Written in STONE

Ethics for the HEART

Written in STONE

Ethics for the HEART

DR. RUBEL SHELLY

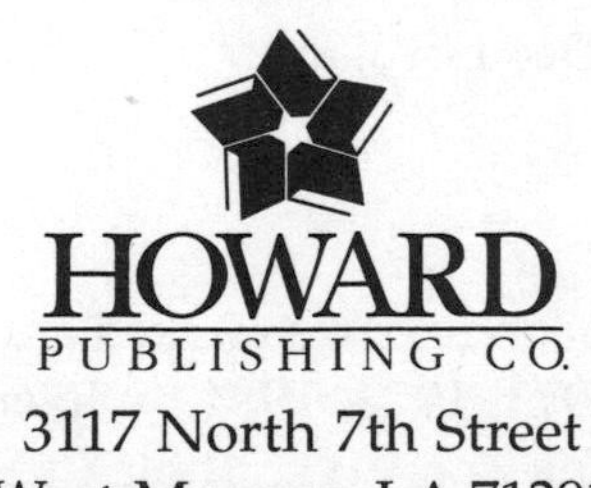

HOWARD
PUBLISHING CO.
3117 North 7th Street
West Monroe, LA 71291

Our purpose at Howard Publishing is:

- *Inspiring* holiness in the lives of believers
- *Instilling* hope in the hearts of struggling people everywhere
- *Instructing* believers toward a deeper faith in Jesus Christ

Because he's coming again

Howard Publishing Co., Inc.
3117 North 7th Street, West Monroe, LA 71291-2227

Written in Stone

Printed in the United States of America
Second printing 1995

Cover Design by LinDee Loveland

ISBN 1-878990-36-5

CONTENTS

INTRODUCTION

Ted Turner, never shy about making his thoughts public, has proposed that we do away with the Ten Commandments. On second thought, that isn't quite right. He actually suggested a rewrite. Setting aside the old, traditional commands about adultery and greed, the media mogul from Atlanta proposes new priorities such as: "I love and respect the planet Earth and all living things thereon, especially my fellow species, mankind"; "I promise to have no more than two children, or no more than my nation suggests"; and "I reject the use of force, particularly military force." Larry King reported his suggestions and said, "Ted Turner's new Ten Commandments make a lot more sense than the old ones."

Not many people feel secure enough to challenge the Decalogue directly. Others of us do so more discreetly—with rationalizations, polite evasions, and covert rebellion. Even some people who consider themselves dedicated Christians somehow think that salvation by grace represents exemption from accountability to divine law.

Marshall Shelley, editor of *Leadership* magazine, tells a wonderful story about an experience he had while studying Hebrew at the University of Denver. His instructor, an Orthodox rabbi, introduced himself as "what you all would call a Pharisee, one who takes God's Law seriously." One evening he lectured on the 613 laws the rabbis have counted in the Torah. For students who were mostly Christian seminarians, he covered Sabbath laws, the dietary laws, and various requirements governing holy days; and he described in detail how Orthodox Jews keep them.

Even some people who consider themselves dedicated Christians somehow think that salvation by grace represents exemption from accountability to divine law.

"I believe that when God speaks, I must obey," said Rabbi Wagner. "Nominal Jews and nominal Christians might disagree with me, but I believe God is a commanding God, that he gives us laws to live by.

"You Christians claim to obey God," he continued. "I've just described the laws of God that I live by. Tell me, you Christians, what laws of God do you obey?"

After an embarrassing silence, Shelley finally responded. "Well, I guess I'd answer the way Jesus did when he was asked to summarize the law. He said to love the Lord your God with all your heart, soul, mind, and strength. And to love your neighbor as yourself."

The rabbi smiled, stroked his beard, and proceeded to tell a story.

"Have you ever heard the story of the centipede with sore feet? He had one hundred feet, and they were all sore. He couldn't walk, so he went to the wisest creature he knew—the owl—to ask what he should do. The owl heard his plight and then intoned his solution: 'Learn to fly, give your feet a rest, and you'll be fine.'

" 'Oh, that's a wonderful idea,' replied the centipede. 'How do I begin?'

"The owl retorted, 'I gave you the principle. The specifics you'll have to work out for yourself.'

"That's what you Christians do," said the rabbi. "You talk about loving God, but how? That's a nice principle, but it's not very practical. It lacks specifics. We Jews like things a little more well-defined."

The rabbi's rebuke is on target for a generation that seems to delight in putting love and law in conflict and in arguing that love may sometimes drive one to break the rules of so absolute a code as the Ten Commandments. Situations are imagined where love is supposed to prompt (perhaps obligate!) ethical persons to steal, lie, or commit adultery.

A biblical view of ethical behavior in general and Christian discipleship in particular correctly recognizes that divine commandments are the only safe guidelines for love. But we don't know the specifics of how to love unless God guides us. Only an omniscient God who knows the end at the beginning could know what is right for us to do under all circumstances. Our limited perspective and piecemeal understanding do not permit us to trust our own judgment in pressure-packed situations.

No one who follows Jesus can legitimately appeal to love as the basis for breaking heaven's rules, for Jesus said, "If you love me, you will obey what I command" (John 14:15). The apostle John underscored this same truth by writing: "This is love for God: to obey his commands" (1 John 5:3).

Need a final word of proof on this from the New Testament? Then hear Paul:

> Let no debt remain outstanding, except the continuing debt to love one another, for he who loves his fellowman has fulfilled the law. The commandments, "Do not commit adultery," "Do not murder," "Do not steal," "Do not covet," and whatever other commandment there may be, are summed up in this one rule: "Love your neighbor as yourself." Love does no harm to its neighbor. Therefore love is the fulfillment of the law. (Rom. 13:8–10)

The permissiveness of modern culture, ethical theory, and theology is an offense against love rather than an authentic application of it. If we love God, we commit to living within his will and honoring his commandments. Love is not an excuse for living outside his will; it is what motivates us to stay within its defined parameters.

No one who follows Jesus can legitimately appeal to love as the basis for breaking heaven's rules.

Love and law are allies, not enemies. Don't let anyone deceive you into thinking you must choose between them. *Law needs love as its driving force,* else it degenerates into cruel legalism. *Love needs law as its eyes,* for it is often blind as to how it should honor or please its object.

In thirteen chapters, this book explores the practical modern consequences of a law code given to Israel through Moses almost 3,500 years ago. Although the singular code, written in stone and known to us as the

Decalogue, was the center of an ancient covenant between Yahweh and Israel, its undergirding principles are eternal and universal and provide ethical standards for the heart. As director Cecil B. deMille observed of the principles established in his classic movie *The Ten Commandments,* "It is impossible for us to break the law. We can only break ourselves against the law."

A foundational definition of an ethical, God-honoring life can best be determined by beginning with the fundamental ten. These commandments, written in stone, have weathered the test of time and continue to speak to our hearts with ethics that provide purpose and guidance for living.

On the morning of the third day there was thunder and lightning, with a thick cloud over the mountain, and a very loud trumpet blast. Everyone in the camp trembled.

Exodus 19:16

CHAPTER ONE

ETHICS GROUNDED IN REVERENCE

The Relationship of God's Person to His Law

Nobody seems to know the difference between right and wrong anymore. What once was nailed down has become loose.

The theme of the '60s was antiestablishment. In protest against government, family, and church, people who had been assured that God was dead sank into a self-destructive era of drugs, uninhibited sex, and moral anarchy. Next we moved into the self-absorbed decade of the '70s. Tom Wolfe dubbed it "The Decade of Me," and its best sellers were *Looking Out for Number One* and *Winning through Intimidation.* Most recently we have endured "The Golden Age of Greed," the decade of the '80s. Athletes gambled on sporting events, Wall Street kingpins were jailed for insider trading, and officials in government were caught in sex, drug, and influence-peddling scandals.

And now in the '90s, we are facing a crisis of ethics. What we once took for granted as "common decency" is now uncommon. The utterly outrageous has become ordinary. The obscene is commonplace. Our code of ethics has eroded on such a massive scale that we have become cynical about morality; and we sense that something is terribly, terribly wrong with the spiritual fabric of our world.

Since 1960, violent crime in America has increased more than 500 percent. A Justice Department study in 1987 predicted that eight out of ten Americans will be victims of violent crime in their lifetimes. Six million violent crimes were recorded by the Justice Department in 1990.

Crime is so prevalent that Americans have altered their lifestyles out of fear. Whole sections of major cities are considered unsafe. One-fourth of the population is estimated to have installed home security systems. Shoppers worry about where to park at shopping malls. Women carry mace in their glove compartments and purses. More and more carry guns. Newspapers and talk shows document the fact that crime is the most important public policy issue in many sections of the country.

As we look to the future, prospects for improvement in the social climate don't look good. Ever since the notorious "wilding" spree of 1989, when a gang of New York City teens raped and beat a woman jogger in Central Park, crimes by adolescents have been getting more notice. Upwards of three million crimes a year are committed in or near the eighty-five thousand public schools in our country. Some inner-city schools have added drive-by-shooting drills to traditional fire drills. Others have fenced-in campuses, metal detectors, and locker searches.

People are wondering aloud about this crisis of ethics and demanding that something be done to reverse the downward spiral. Will the twenty-first century witness a renewed sensitivity to fundamental morality? Will honesty, kindness, courage, justice, and self-discipline reemerge? Or will we only cluck our tongues and continue to commit moral suicide?

WE DID IT TO OURSELVES

We Lost Our Sensitivity

Remember the old story about the frog in a pan of water on the stove? The temperature was raised so gradually that he was insensitive to the change. He was finally cooked without ever trying to escape. Over the past few decades, our incremental acceptance of obscenity and violence has elevated our tolerance for evil. As the words and pictures around us have gradually become more graphic, bizarre, and corrupt, we have become desensitized. And with the numbing of our moral sensitivities has come not only greater tolerance for, but also increased involvement with, moral impurity.

We Gave Up Our Voice

While the temperature of immorality has gradually escalated, religion, believers, and evangelists have failed us. In general, religion has been in retreat. Instead of engagement and prophetic challenge, religion has offered Marxist theology, ordination of homosexuals, and wholesale mutilation of Scripture. Believers have been crippled by intimidation: some have been so concerned about sophistication or so fearful of being criticized for Bible-based values that they have been tolerant when they should have been outraged, indulgent when they ought to have been indignant. Some of the best-known evangelists have either been defrocked for their immoralities or put in jail for their crimes. These haven't been the best of times for people who are supposed to uphold righteousness and honor the name of the Almighty.

With the numbing of our moral sensitivities has come not only greater tolerance for, but also increased involvement with, moral impurity.

Too often, the only voices speaking for principles and human dignity have been secular opinion leaders. Addressing the graduating class at Duke University in 1987, ABC's Ted Koppel said:

> Our society finds truth too strong a medicine to digest undiluted. In its purest form, truth is not a polite tap on the shoulder. It is a howling reproach. What Moses brought down from Mt. Sinai were not the Ten Suggestions. They are commandments. Are, not were. The sheer brilliance of the Ten Commandments is that they codify in a handful of words acceptable human behavior, not just for then or now, but for all time.

If it seems strange that a widely heard—and, it should be added, widely criticized—call for recognition of the Ten Commandments should come from the anchor of television's *Nightline* rather than from a respected and influential church leader, it shouldn't. While discussions of ethics are very much in vogue in the '90s, religious personnel are not. Our society views *ethics* as an acceptable topic for discussion, but *Scripture* is not regarded with the same respect. Most professional schools have required ethics courses in their curricula—business ethics, medical ethics, legal ethics, etc.—but Scripture is not considered in these seminars, university courses, and newspaper columns. We are part of a culture where personal religion as the rule of private conduct is praised but where the Bible as a relevant standard for public life is discounted. It is therefore deemed appropriate for a Christian to speak from a pulpit to teach personal piety or personal salvation, but it is judged unacceptable by many for that same Christian to speak in the university, newspaper, evening news, or other public forums about social issues or public policy.

Perhaps Christians have retreated from dialogue with the public sector because of a fundamental fear that we no longer share common ground with our unbelieving neighbors.

THE NATURE OF MORALITY

Morality Begins with God

For Christians, *all morality begins with the person and nature of God.* Before discussions of principle or law must come worship of the Creator. The study of *Christian* ethics begins, therefore, with an awareness of the personal presence of God.

There were many options open to Yahweh for the giving of the Ten Commandments. Why did he reveal himself to the people of Israel by the thunder, lightning, and a loud trumpet call at Sinai? Surely it was to establish the relationship in their minds between his *person* and his *law.* The cloud, thunder, and lightning that signaled God's presence made the encamped nation of Israel "tremble" before him. In a posture of reverence, they were able to receive covenant words. The abiding memory of that event called them to keep the words of the Law. It was as if he wanted them to understand that obedience to law must grow out of some underlying tie between the lawgiver and would-be lawkeepers.

Jesus would develop this theme during his personal ministry by saying, "If you love me, you will obey what I command" (John 14:15). Thus, law is not the basis for comprehending or encountering God; it is the guideline for discipleship among people who have been sought and confronted by him.

As a discipline, *ethics* is an inquiry into the nature of right and wrong, good conduct and bad. It seeks to define and articulate the moral life. Understanding from Jesus Christ that the two great commandments are love for God and love for neighbor (Matt. 22:34–40), Christian ethics seek to flesh out the practical demands of these two underlying commands for daily life.

Legalism Versus Antinomianism

The history of the Christian church shows that we have not done well either in formulating an ethical theory or in living ethical lives. On the one hand, there have been people and periods notorious for their concern to pore over, codify, and enforce laws derived from Scripture; on the other, there have been intervals and persons celebrated for their contrived reading of Paul's statement "for freedom Christ has set us free" and their resulting repudiation of all rules and doctrines. The former is legalism; the latter is antinomianism.

Legalism, whether ancient or modern, attempts to focus the will of God into a simplistic formulation of rules to govern any and all situations. Thus the ancient Pharisees debated the meaning of the words of the Torah and deduced from them a regulation for every contingency. The result was what Peter once termed "a yoke that neither we nor our fathers have been able to bear" (Acts 15:10b).

Antinomianism, by contrast, sets aside all rules and laws as sub-Christian. It argues for the right of each person to confront every new life-situation in radical freedom and to decide only then the God-honoring thing to do. Joseph Fletcher's contextual approach to ethics in his famous book, *Situation Ethics,* is a case in point of this approach to ethical theory.

Legalism does not understand the nature of divine commands, refuses to face the complexity of many ethical dilemmas, and waives any primary obligation for showing compassion. Antinomianism, on the other hand, tends to set aside all moral instruction in favor of well-intentioned subjectivism. While the Bible contains no direct data about genetic engineering, *in vitro* fertilization, euthanasia, or any number of modern complexities, Scripture does offer principles on which to base our ethical choices. The lone decision maker would have to be God himself in order to understand the endless contingencies involved in each setting of moral choice and to make responsible decisions. The truth must lie some place other than in these two extremes.

The Nature of Deity Defines Morality

An action is right not because God has willed it so but because it corresponds to and exemplifies his nature. A behavior is wrong not because of some whimsical decision of God but because it is inconsistent with his perfect goodness. For example, God could neither lie nor decree that lying is right, for truth is fundamental to his being (John 3:33; Rom. 3:4). Telling the truth corresponds to the nature of God and is therefore a righteous act. Lying is contrary, not merely to God's law, but to his being.

An action is right not because God has willed it so but because it corresponds to and exemplifies his nature.

The Relevance of Scripture

Christian ethics can never ignore Scripture. Since we believe that the writers of both Old and New Testaments were moved by the Spirit of God (2 Pet. 1:20–21), what they said must be normative for us. At the same time, however, we freely grant that the fullest revelation of God was not in words but in a person—Jesus of Nazareth. On occasion we watch in awe as he deals with moral dilemmas growing out of the Law of Moses: working to meet human need on the Sabbath (Mark 2:23–28; Luke 13:10–17), balancing judgment and mercy (John 8:11), challenging the human tendency to substitute ritual for compassion (Matt. 23:16–24), etc.

So, while granting that some laws of Scripture are culture-specific to a time and place other than our own, Christians still affirm that the words of the Bible are perpetually relevant. For example, our urban society neither allows nor obliges us to harvest fields so as to leave the edges for the poor—as did the Old Testament Jewish society (Lev. 19:9–10)—but we are under perpetual obligation to find appropriate ways to help the poorest and weakest among us.

Apart from the perfection of God as witnessed in Jesus Christ, goodness is a mere nonsense word that has no meaningful place in discourse about human behavior. Ethicists divorced from the specific revelation of the Bible argue endlessly over the meaning of the terms right and wrong. But in light of Scripture's teachings as personified in Jesus, these words have genuine substance.

God in Us

Even the person who says he or she does not believe in God derives his or her every notion of right conduct from the Creator. All people have an intuitive moral sense because they are created in the image of God. Paul insisted that pagans "show that the requirements of the law are written on their hearts, their consciences also bearing witness, and their thoughts now accusing, now even defending them" (Rom. 2:15). Why does an atheist cry out against social injustice? Why does an unbeliever sign petitions against child pornography in her city? It is because God has created everyone with an innate sense of moral obligation.

To inform this innate sense, God has revealed himself in human history. As we receive his revelation—through conscience, Scripture, and Jesus—we receive guidance in knowing the will of God. As we receive strength from the Holy Spirit, our wills are empowered to live to his glory in righteousness. As God develops ethical character in us through this process, a genuine purity of heart emerges that allows us simultaneously to live under law and to imitate the example of Jesus in balancing the competing claims of even the most complex of moral dilemmas. Rather than using rules to selfish advantage (cf. Matt. 23:1 ff.), we learn to apply them with fairness, respect for the dignity of all parties concerned, and compassion.

THE OLD TESTAMENT REVEALS AN ETERNAL MORAL CODE

The Bible is a *progressive revelation* of the will of God. That is to say, it is the gradual unfolding of the body of truth God has revealed to humankind. From Adam to Noah to Abraham to Moses to Jesus, more and more of the revelation of heaven was given. At different times and in a variety of ways, God addressed himself to his human creatures. This process reached its zenith in Jesus (Heb. 1:1–2).

When we speak of revelation as "progressive" in nature, we should be careful to define our meaning. There was no evolutionary progress toward truth by a trial-and-error method. All the prophets chosen by God to be part of the revelatory process—in both the Old and New Testaments—were equally moved by the Spirit. What each said was true, spiritual, and elevating. The progression in the process was from *partial to complete,* not from *error to truth.*

While the types and shadows of the Old Testament doctrine of atonement (animal sacrifice) have given way to the reality of redemption in Christ (his once-for-all sacrifice on the cross), the basic ethical teachings of the Old Testament do reflect an eternally correct moral code. While the Old Testament is not the covenant by which people living today will ultimately be judged, it does provide basic insight into the moral will of God and is valuable for our ongoing spiritual instruction (Rom. 15:4).

Many of the most basic moral principles were given from the start. Take, for example, what Genesis 2:24 teaches about the one-man-one-woman-for-life nature of marriage. "For this reason a man will leave his father and mother and be united to his wife, and they will become one flesh." Jesus would later cite this very text (Matt. 19:4–5) as a rebuke to the widespread disregard for the sacredness of marriage in his time: it was "hardness of heart" that caused men to abandon its original inviolability (Matt. 19:8). As another example, consider what God told Noah about the worth of human life. "Whoever sheds the blood of man, by man shall his blood be shed; for in the image of God has God made man" (Gen. 9:6). Murder is wrong because every human being of whatever race, sex, or language bears God's own image. This is a foundation principle of biblical ethics.

In the Ten Commandments, one finds the most succinct statement of human responsibility ever given. The Decalogue was at the heart of ancient Israel's duties to God and humanity. More than that, it remains the basic moral framework within which men and women of all generations are expected to live.

Three thousand five hundred years ago, Yahweh delivered the Hebrew nation from captivity in Egypt. Around 1450 B.C. (cf. 1 Kings 6:1), a nation of more than two million souls left Egypt under the leadership of Moses. Their exodus was the beginning of a perilous journey to a promised land. The pivotal event at the start of this experience was the establishment of a covenant between Yahweh and Israel at Mount Sinai.

Approximately three months after the Exodus, Moses and the people arrived at the base of the mountain. According to Exodus 19:1–8, they camped there for a full year to receive and learn the provisions of the covenant God was making with them. Although this covenant was, for the Jewish people (Exod. 34:27–28), temporary (Jer. 31:31–34) and brought to fulfillment in Jesus (Gal. 3:24–25), the spiritual and moral insights embodied in it are eternal.

CONCLUSION

The goal of this book is to pursue a theological and practical study of the Decalogue. Although the Bible has scores and even hundreds of particular commands that relate to spiritual and ethical life, the Ten Commandments are the starting point for serious study of ethical questions. They are not an end in themselves; indeed, their end, or goal, is to bring us to Jesus Christ. Law cannot save, but it can make us sense our need for a Savior.

Ted Koppel said of the Ten Commandments: "There is harmony and inner peace to be found in following a moral compass that points in the same direction regardless of fashion or trend." Our world's need for such a compass is evident, and a reverent study of the Decalogue can only bring benefit to all who participate in it.

From the very beginning, however, we must understand that ethics is a way of seeing God and ourselves in relation to him before it is a matter of behaving a certain way. Without a vision of God as high, lifted up, and worthy of worship, there will be no permanent change of life. Surely that is why God produced such a dramatic scene on Mount Sinai.

Shouting commandments and threats at people will not produce change. Change begins with the vision of God. And that vision can only come today through a faithful, countercultural church. A faithful church must take holiness seriously—without being self-righteous. It must preach Jesus by both deeds and words—without presuming to substitute the latter for the former. It must be a conscience to the world—without being strident or harsh.

Worship is the foundation on which the ethical life of the people of God is built. Until we feel the "tremble" produced by a vision of God's glory and might, making ethical choices is a burdensome duty. But when ethics are grounded in reverence, the pursuit of a holy lifestyle becomes the joyous enterprise of discipleship.

QUESTIONS FOR ADDITIONAL REFLECTION

1. Can you recall situations in which you should have spoken out against wrong rather than keeping silent? How can one "speak the truth in love" when God's law is being ignored?

2. What is the Christian's role in public life? Should religion remain strictly private, or does it have implications for the public arena? If it has public implications, to what extent?

3. Do you understand the claim of this chapter that ethical standards for a Christian are based in the person and nature of God? Are you conscious of this fact in your personal morality?

4. Describe a particular biblical text, story, or experience that you believe most clearly reveals God's holy nature to you.

5. If *legalism* is a one and *antinomianism* is a ten, where are you in that range today? Where were you five or ten years ago? Where do you see yourself ten years from now? Explore your journey in this area.

6. How do you resolve ethical questions about genetic engineering, euthanasia, *in vitro* fertilization, etc.? What are some other contemporary ethical questions that the Bible does not answer directly?

7. How do we determine which laws of Scripture are culturally specific? What guidelines can we use to find their present relevance?

8. Are you conscious of God's Spirit having helped you to develop the purity of heart that allows you to imitate Christ? How has the process worked in your life?

9. Do you understand ethics as a way of *seeing* or *acting?* How are the two different? How are they related?

I am the L*ORD*
your God, who
brought you
out of Egypt,
out of the land
of slavery.

Exodus 20:2

CHAPTER TWO

THE INSEPARABLE BOND OF LAW TO GRACE

Grace as the Background for Divine Law

The recitation or study of the Ten Commandments typically begins with Exodus 20:3. It is a serious oversight, however, to ignore the words Yahweh spoke as a preamble to the core laws that would serve as the basis for religion and morality in Israel: "I am the LORD your God, who brought you out of Egypt, out of the land of slavery." Before listing the "must-dos" of the people, there was a reminder of the "already-done" by God. Thus does the Decalogue affirm the inseparable relationship of law to grace within Judeo-Christian faith. From the beginning, *grace* has been the background for divine *law.*

DELIVERANCE ALWAYS PRECEDES OBEDIENCE

Israel's obedience to divine law was not the basis of that nation's deliverance. It was exactly the reverse.

Deliverance by the mighty hand of God provided freedom to more than two million souls. In their freedom, they were called to be holy, obedient, and righteous. The *chronology* of events cannot be debated: the good news of deliverance came prior to the law. Neither can the *theology* of biblical faith be debated: the Good News of deliverance comes before our duties to or performance under the law. Gospel before demand, grace before law, God's good deed before human good deeds—the order of things is constant and essential in biblical theology.

Gospel before demand, grace before law—the order of things is constant and essential in biblical theology.

THE TWO EXTREMES: LEGALISM AND UNIVERSALISM

Instead of following God's order, however, our tendency is to move toward one of two extremes. One human inclination is to reverse God's order and place law before grace. This propensity is described as *legalism* (the belief that salvation is based on ability to keep law). Legalism sees law as the means to receiving grace and tries to put human deeds of obedience prior to God's work of grace. But this tendency raises fundamental questions regarding the nature and purpose of law: Is law the means of getting to God? Does our obedience to law make us righteous before God? The Bible answers these questions with a resounding negative:

"Therefore no one will be declared righteous in [God's] sight by observing the law" (Rom. 3:20a).

Another human propensity that must be curbed is toward universalism (the belief that all are saved because of God's gracious nature). This tendency exhibits itself in impurity, license, and rebellion. But a holy God will not be mocked by his creatures. In spite of his loving nature, people who defy God in order to satisfy their corrupt desires will have no part in the kingdom of God (Gal. 5:19–21).

What, then, is the truth of the matter? Are we reduced to a choice between universalism and legalism? Biblical religion offers a third alternative: trusting obedience.

TRUSTING OBEDIENCE

Illustrated by the Example of Abraham

For both Jews and Christians, Abraham is offered as the paradigm of salvation by faith. We are to learn from his experience and follow his example. Here is what Paul said of his salvation:

> It was not through law that Abraham and his offspring received the promise that he would be heir of the world, but through the righteousness that comes by faith. For if those who live by law are heirs, faith has no value and the promise is worthless, because law brings wrath. And where there is no law there is no transgression.
>
> Therefore, the promise comes by faith, so that it may be by grace and may be guaranteed to all Abraham's offspring—not only to those who are of the law but also to those who are of the faith of Abraham. He is the father of us all. (Rom. 4:13–16; cf. 4:1–5)

To make human activity under law the ground of deliverance from bondage flies in the face of all that the Bible teaches about salvation.

At the same time, the Bible is equally emphatic about the necessity of a faith that is alive, active, and obedient to God. Thus the half-brother of Jesus also appealed to the Abraham story:

> You foolish man, do you want evidence that faith without deeds is useless? Was not our ancestor Abraham considered righteous for what he did when he offered his son Isaac on the altar? You see that his faith and his actions were working together, and his faith was made complete by what he did. And the scripture was fulfilled that says, "Abraham believed God, and it was credited to him as righteousness," and he was called God's friend. You see that a person is justified by what he does and not by faith alone. (James 2:20–24)

Looking closely at Abraham as a case study, we see that the initiative for all that happened in his role as "father of the faithful" was with God. By a sovereign act of grace, God chose and called Abraham. The idea of leaving Ur didn't originate with Abraham. When he left that ancient city, he hadn't figured out where to go. Instead, he trusted God and followed his leading. When the process ended, all the glory belonged to God rather than Abraham. Yet God had not achieved his purpose in the ancient patriarch's life against Abraham's will.

> By faith Abraham, when called to go to a place he would later receive as his inheritance, obeyed and went, even though he did not know where he was going. By faith he made his home in the promised land like a stranger in a foreign country; he lived in tents, as did Isaac and Jacob, who were heirs with him of the same promise. For he was looking forward to the city with foundations, whose architect and builder is God. (Heb. 11:8–10)

The "because of" to Abraham's story was God. All the wonderful things that came to him and his descendants were because of God's choice, God's grace, and God's faithfulness. In a very real sense, Abraham contributed nothing to the drama and was even unnecessary to it. God could have accomplished his purpose through another person and in some other manner. The only thing that can be considered his "contribution" was his willingness to be included in God's purpose. He so trusted Yahweh that he accepted his call and obeyed his instructions. Along the way, he lied (Gen. 12:10–20; cf. 20:1 ff.), his faith failed (Gen. 17:17), and his full humanity was otherwise displayed. But God remained faithful.

Illustrated by the History of Israel

Turning now to the experience of Abraham's descendants in Egypt, does anyone who knows the Bible story believe Israel delivered itself from bondage? Of course not. The Exodus was a mighty display of God's power in the midst of Israel's weakness. God forced Pharaoh's hand and made him release an enslaved people. On the other hand, does anyone believe that God would have protected an Israelite who was outside a blood-protected house from death on the night of the Exodus? Does anyone seriously think that a lazy Hebrew who stayed behind on that fateful night would have escaped harm at the hands of the Egyptians who found him the next day? Of course not. God's mighty act of deliverance did not force freedom on people who had no interest in it. It placed release from bondage within their grasp and gave them the choice of accepting or rejecting it.

As their forefather Abraham, the Israelites had to demonstrate their faith by moving out on God's call.

Their faith had to show itself in killing the lamb, putting its blood on the door, and waiting in the blood-marked houses until the signal to leave was given. With this act of deliverance as background, the Decalogue was given as still another expression of God's grace to the people of Israel.

The Ten Commandments are more correctly understood as the "must-dos" for a faith community that was formed by the "already-done" divine act of liberation from slavery.

It would be altogether wrong-headed to see the Ten Commandments as somehow contradictory to God's grace. It would be equally wrong to see them as a ten-runged ladder to enable people to enter a grace relationship with God. They are more correctly understood as the "must-dos" for a faith community that was formed by the "already-done" divine act of liberation from slavery.

WHAT DIFFERENCE DOES IT MAKE?

From past experience, I can imagine someone saying at this point: "I don't see the point of all this. What difference does it make anyway? There's law and grace, and we have to deal with both to be faithful to God." But getting things right about the relationship of the two makes all the difference in the world.

Teaching Obedience before Deliverance Produces Failure

As a preacher, I have seen too many people turn back who once had walked with the Lord. Some who were active and dedicated believers have become careless and apathetic Christians. Some have become apostates. I am convinced that many of these cases are the result of poor teaching about the basis of our relationship with God.

Too often we teach the gospel this way: "Friend, your life is messed up because of sin; you need to read the Bible, do what it says, and find the joy of a new way of living." But this is the wrong way to go about it. Teaching people to obey the Bible's rules in order to find deliverance and peace is exactly backward to the biblical method. The Gospel message begins with the declaration of what God has done to set us free. Then, as we respond, God matures us into worship, understanding of the will of God, and fruitful obedience.

A girl I knew growing up had to endure a home and church that demanded more of her than she—or anyone else—could give. Her father demanded perfect grades and perfect behavior. Her preacher taught her that God demanded perfect theology and perfect performance. She lived in fear of failing or disappointing. She got the message that acceptance was based on achievement. Failure would mean certain rejection. So when her marriage failed, her world collapsed. Emotionally and spiritually, this woman, who had been programmed to see herself as unworthy of love and always teetering on the brink of rejection, broke under the weight. Does anyone wonder why?

The Gospel is the wonderful news of acceptance through Christ rather than through accomplishment. It must always be presented as a free gift and never as a series of hurdles to clear.

It doesn't take a genius to discover that something is terribly and devastatingly wrong on Planet Earth. We continue producing the likes of Pol Pot, Idi Amin, and Saddam Hussein. Our political systems create apartheid and totalitarian rule. Self-indulgent materialism, chemical dependency, and sexual immorality destroy whole families.

At the most personal level, people are frustrated and lonely. Millions have no goal for their lives. They can't relate to one another, don't keep promises, and wonder aloud why they aren't happy. Marriages fail. Parents and children don't speak to one another. Adults cry themselves to sleep and wish they could die. Something is dreadfully wrong.

Burdened to remedy our world, we discover divine laws in the Ten Commandments or Sermon on the Mount. We begin to obey them and press them on others. Sure enough, the situation begins to improve. But with every disobedience comes guilt. Then there is struggle, followed by tiredness. Shame sets in. Then come more failures and increasing shame. Then come collapse, deliberate disobedience, and rejection of the law that initially seemed so promising and helpful. And thus has come about the sad, dispirited faith of some and the outright apostasy of others. And people who taught those poor souls a backward approach to salvation have set them up to fail. They surely didn't mean to, but they did. Paul's words already quoted once in this chapter must be repeated again here: "Therefore no one will be declared righteous in his sight by observing the law; rather, through the law we become conscious of sin" (Rom. 3:20).

Understanding Deliverance Produces Obedience

God's scheme of redemption does not call for us to put things right in our world on the basis of rules. To the contrary, it calls for us to leave the initiative with him and to trust his ability to do everything necessary to save us. He doesn't need our help. And trying to lend a hand will only ruin his scheme.

> But now a righteousness from God, apart from law, has been made known, to which the Law and the Prophets testify. This righteousness from God comes through faith in Jesus Christ to all who believe. (Rom. 3:21–22)

God's way starts with love. From his wonderful love come mighty acts of deliverance from slavery. This, in turn, gives personal peace. But then, strangely enough, comes a sense of guilt—arising both from one's sense of unworthiness and instances of personal failure. So God gives more forgiveness. Then worship and joy follow. And through a process of patient nurturing, faithfulness results.

Strange as it may sound, attempts at justification through law invariably lead to disobedience and failure. Understanding that salvation is by grace produces obedience and faithfulness. This contrast is so radical to our human approach to making things right that most reject it. Only an understanding that salvation is by grace puts law in its rightful place and enables the seeking soul to rejoice in redemption and to honor the demands of law in her life.

In summarizing what he was about to do for the enslaved Israelites, Yahweh told Moses:

> I have indeed seen the misery of my people in Egypt. I have heard them crying out because of their slave drivers, and I am concerned about their suffering. So I

> have come down to rescue them from the hand of the Egyptians and to bring them up out of that land into a good and spacious land, a land flowing with milk and honey. (Exod. 3:7–8)

Entering a covenant relationship with the nation at Mount Sinai and teaching them of his holiness through the Ten Commandments would come *after* a powerful deliverance.

Grace Does Not Exclude Obligation

Any believer's personal experience of salvation begins with deliverance. Salvation then moves the individual to more study, greater awareness of spiritual duties, and a growing desire to honor God in the fulfillment of those duties. John Wesley expressed it this way: "The nature of the covenant of grace gives you no ground, no encouragement at all, to set aside any instance or degree of obedience, any part or measure of holiness." Begin with the imposition of duties as the means to grace, however, and you have substituted a cruel legalism for the liberating message of the gospel.

Consistent with the statement from Wesley, it probably needs to be stressed that grace does not free one from obligation. Indeed, too many people are eager to heed the call of grace without heeding the call to holiness. They embrace a form of religion that is sufficient to mitigate their guilt but inadequate to give purpose to their lives. They sit in church pews, sing the songs of faith, and then return to a world where God has no meaningful place. He is called on to dispense occasional forgiveness in the face of a "major" transgression, but he is not sovereign in daily experience. This is a travesty against grace. It is what Dietrich Bonhoeffer called "cheap grace."

God's mighty acts in history have not resulted in salvation for everyone. In spite of his amazing grace, many will be lost for eternity (Matt. 7:21–23; 25:31–46). Human responsibility to God is an important aspect of our relationship with him.

Too many people embrace a form of religion that is sufficient to mitigate their guilt but inadequate to give purpose to their lives.

With Israel at Mount Sinai and with today's church, *discipleship* is the desired outcome of grace lavishly bestowed.

HOW TO USE THE DECALOGUE

The remaining chapters of this book will look at each of the ten commandments in sequence. In order to avoid misappropriating the Ten Commandments, we must be very clear about how we use them. There are three legitimate expectations we may bring to our upcoming studies.

First, these commandments reflect divine ideals for human behavior. Do you want to know how God feels about lying or stealing? Read the Ten Commandments. Do you want to know how seriously heaven regards adultery? Read the Ten Commandments. Although Jesus came to "fulfill" the Law of Moses, he did not come to renounce Moses or to disown the Ten Commandments. As a matter of fact, the Son of God upheld everything taught in the Law about humanity's fundamental religious and ethical duties. In fulfilling the types and shadows of the old covenant, he affirmed every insight found in the Decalogue and disclaimed none.

While using them as divine ideals and norms, we must be careful not to interpret these laws as boundaries to divine love. God loves us even when we break his commandments and fall short of his ideal for our lives. Not only do we need to remember that for our own sakes but also for the sake of the way we treat the people around us.

Second, the Ten Commandments serve to mark the trouble spots of life. Learning where those snares are can save us an abundance of unnecessary grief and heartache. In *To My People with Love,* John Killinger writes:

> In her beautiful novel about Maine, *The Country of the Pointed Firs,* Sara Orne Jewett describes the ascent of a woman writer on the pathway leading to the home of a retired sea captain named Elijah Tilley.
>
> On the way, the woman notes a number of stakes randomly scattered about the property, with no discernible order. Each is painted white and trimmed in yellow, like the captain's house. Curious, she asks Captain Tilley what they mean. When he first plowed the ground, he says, his plow snagged on many large rocks just beneath the surface. So he set out the stakes where the rocks lay in order to avoid them in the future.
>
> In a sense, this is what God has done with the Ten Commandments. . . . He has said, "These are the trouble spots in life. Avoid these, and you won't snag your plow."

Third, although law cannot save us, it can bring us to Christ for salvation. "So the law was put in charge to lead us to Christ that we might be justified by faith" (Gal. 3:24).

It is our inability to keep any law adequately—including but not limited to the Ten Commandments—that makes us realize how necessary the saving work of Christ is. Apart from him, we have no hope.

CONCLUSION

Several times in this chapter, Paul has been quoted on the subject of law and grace. The reason he wrote so much about this theme is rooted in his own experience. Early in his spiritual life, he understood God as a critic of human behavior who laid down unyielding rules and standards for his obedience. Because of this, Paul believed he was obligated to live up to the demands of law in order to escape punishment as a lawbreaker. Paul expected to be saved only if he could prove himself righteous under law.

But it wasn't working for him. He knew the commands, but he could not keep pace with their flawless expectations. The very things he said he would do, often went undone; and the commands he tried hardest not to break were the ones he violated most often. It was hopeless for *Paul the legalist*.

Then came the Damascus Road and an encounter with Jesus. Paul's entire life was turned around. He came to believe that the very law he had been unable to honor perfectly had been kept flawlessly by Jesus, who then offered himself as Paul's substitute and died in his place. The right standing with God that Paul had been pursuing through law was now his on the basis of Christ's work on his behalf. What he could not achieve under law, he accepted on the basis of grace.

Until this good day, though, many of us act like scared mice before a cosmic cat. We resent rules that we try, with mounting frustration, to keep. Defensive before the letter of the law, we miss its spirit altogether. Trying to live up to our duties in order to escape punishment, we judge both ourselves and others unmercifully.

What Paul learned then is still true now. It has always been true. God has never worked any other way in rescuing and redeeming his people. Abraham, Israel, Paul, you—all are offered a relationship by grace that cannot be attained under law.

From the beginning, then, let's get it straight. It is grace before law, gospel before demand, justification before sanctification. Deliverance from Pharaoh, alcohol, homosexuality, or any other form of slavery originates in grace. You accept your freedom through faith and can never earn it through personal accomplishment under law. Out of gratitude for deliverance, you will learn respect for every divine commandment and grow in your ability to honor the holy expectations embodied in them.

When you are safely home in heaven, you will neither boast of your accomplishments nor receive plaudits for your ability to keep rules. You will praise God for his grace. Getting that fixed in your mind and acting accordingly will make life better for you. The difference in the two approaches is the difference between guilt and pardon, severity and mercy, death and life.

QUESTIONS FOR ADDITIONAL REFLECTION

1. Have you ever tried using law to get into relationship with God? How? What was the result?
2. Are you more inclined to be a legalist or a universalist? Why? Which is the worse error? Why?
3. Has God ever called you to "leave Ur"? If so, how did you respond? How did God respond? Reflect on some specific ways God has asked you to demonstrate your faith.
4. Under what circumstances does obedience to the divine will produce peace and joy? Have you ever tried to share this insight with someone else? What was her or his response?
5. What keeps us from presenting the gospel as a gift? Why do we tend to include so many hurdles?
6. Have you ever used grace as an excuse to refuse obedience to God? What was the result?
7. Why does legalism inevitably lead to disobedience and failure? Is this true for every area of life (e.g., marriage, child-rearing, work) or only in one's relationship with God?
8. Do you have trouble reflecting God's love for those who break his commandments in your sphere of acquaintance? Explain your answer.
9. Have you ever "hit a rock" in your life where God has put up a marker? What were the consequences for you? For others who are important to you?
10. Has law helped bring you to Christ? How?

You shall have no other gods before me.

Exodus 20:3

CHAPTER THREE

GOD AS CENTER AND CIRCUMFERENCE

1

"You shall have no other gods before me."

The first commandment not only comes at the head of the list of ten but is the prerequisite worldview for making sense of the nine to follow. If God is truly God, all that he speaks is true and every commandment from him must be obeyed. If God is truly God, there is no person or power that can defeat his purposes. If God is truly God, all who belong to him are safe beyond anyone's power to crush them.

Biblical religion is *exclusive* in nature. The God who revealed himself by the covenant name Yahweh to Israel and who became flesh in the person of Jesus of Nazareth will not accept a place in the pantheon of gods. He alone is divine and claims the right to be both center and circumference to human belief, values, and behavior.

To make God the *center* of one's life is to focus heart, soul, mind, and strength on him; it is to be deeply in love with one's creator and redeemer. To make God the *circumference* of one's life is to adopt the lifestyle of a dedicated disciple; it is to know, affirm, and live within the parameters of heaven's revealed will.

Biblical religion is exclusive in nature.

In Kyoto, Japan, there is reported to be a place of worship called the Temple of the Thousand Buddhas. Inside the shrine are more than a thousand likenesses of the Buddha, each a little different from every other. Supposedly they are there so a worshiper can enter, find the one that looks most like himself, and worship it. Humans look for a god in their own image, but Judeo-Christian theology repudiates anthropocentric (man-centered) religion in favor of theocentric (God-centered) faith.

In the case of Judaism, think of the words of the ancient *Shema:* "Hear, O Israel: The LORD our God, the LORD is one. Love the LORD your God with all your heart and with all your soul and with all your strength" (Deut. 6:4–5; cf. Matt. 22:37–38). If the entirety of one's being is given to the love of Yahweh, there is no place for another deity. With heart, soul, and strength given to him, all the devotee's life is offered as a living sacrifice to God.

When Jesus came on the scene, he both identified himself with Yahweh of the Old Testament and claimed the same exclusive role in his disciples' faith that Yahweh had claimed within Israel. "I am the way and the truth and the life," he said. "No one comes to the Father except through me" (John 14:6). Thus the early church preached: "Salvation is found in no one else, for there is no other name under heaven given to men by which we must be saved" (Acts 4:12).

Such an uncompromising claim is too strong for many today. "It is all right for you to believe whatever you wish about Jesus," they say, "but that is only your truth and may not be appropriate for someone else." Although we are accustomed to such a view, that sort of language sounds preposterous if put in the mouth of a prophet or apostle. Can you imagine Moses saying to Pharaoh, "You may not know the name of our God, Yahweh, and I understand and respect your devotion to Ra; but perhaps we could discuss freedom of religion for your Hebrew subjects"? Or can you imagine Paul telling Agrippa, "Oh, sir, you misunderstood the point of my speech. I was simply testifying as to my experience of Jesus and had no intent of trying to 'proselyte' you to *my* personal faith"?

A *Sports Illustrated* columnist complained in February 1991 about athletes going public with their faith. While saying he was willing to "put up with" an occasional "Thank the Lord," the writer said he was offended by the sight of professional athletes from opposing teams huddling after the game to pray in public view. "Athletes are entitled to freedom of religion like anyone else," he wrote, "but let them exercise it on their own time." People who say such things don't understand that Christian faith was never meant to be limited to a believer's "own time" but must overflow into everything he or she does. Though intensely personal, biblical faith is *not* private.

In this chapter, we will examine the pagan view of God—which, whether ancient or modern, is very different from the biblical view. We will next explore the legitimacy of the Christian's "intolerant" posture toward other deities and religious systems. Then we will point out some practical implications of the view of human life that make God both center and circumference of one's existence.

A PAGAN VIEW OF DEITY

When most of us hear the word *paganism,* we think of bygone days of superstition, witchcraft, and bizarre ritual. Our minds go back to the Babylonians or Greeks. Such terms as *polytheism* or *pantheism* flash into consciousness. We may even conjure up images of human sacrifice.

The truth of the matter is, however, that pagan ideas are not confined to times of the distant past. The so-called New Age Movement is merely a commercially successful form of ancient delusions about reincarnation, communication with the dead, and magical charms.

Paganism in all its forms has some common themes. *First,* the pagan worldview holds that reality is continuous and ultimately unbounded. "All is one" goes the chant, meaning that any apparent distinctions between rocks, squirrels, women, or God are only illusory and not real. This is a form of philosophical monism (a view that all existence reduces to a single order of reality) and amounts to pantheism revived. *Second,* it asserts that we are all divine and destined for union with the One. *Third,* paganism holds that self-fulfillment is the ultimate good for any one of us. *Fourth,* it insists that there are as many realities and truths as there are people to create their own realities and truths and that no reality has any greater value or legitimacy than any other. *Fifth,* paganism believes that all religions are one. Buddhists and Christians and atheists, according to pagan cults, are equally right and equally wrong in their attempts to discover truth. Ultimately, we will all be absorbed at some point into the One and know peace.

From this thumbnail sketch of pagan religions, it is not hard to comprehend why the Decalogue's "You shall have no other gods before me" comes as such a bombshell. The Ten Commandments do not embrace an inclusivism that sees all religion as fundamentally the same and all so-called gods as equally worthy of veneration.

During the time of Hebrew captivity in Egypt, the Jews were surrounded by the beliefs and trappings of paganism. The Egyptians worshiped river and land, cattle and sun, fate and Pharaoh. In the sequence of plagues brought against them, Israel's God showed that the Egyptian deities of land, sky, and water could not withstand his power. In the final plague, even the "divine" Pharaoh's house was invaded by death when his firstborn son died. By this display of might, Yahweh not only struck a blow against what was false but also claimed his rightful place in the hearts of the Hebrew people.

Although they had retained their identity in Egypt, it is unlikely that the Israelites remained unaffected by the paganism around them. What did it say to most people, after all, that Yahweh's people were enslaved by the followers of the gods of Egypt? Thus, when the time was right, Israel's God acted on their behalf. He showed himself to be a compassionate redeemer who would tolerate no rival. With the people at the base of Mount Sinai, he affirmed his love and demanded that his covenant people give him their undivided allegiance.

GOD'S RIGHT TO REIGN

In the name of tolerance or pluralism, our culture treats all points of view as equally legitimate and treats differences of belief and values as unimportant. But there is a vast difference between *tolerance* in a pluralistic society and *syncretism* in religion. I affirm the need for a tolerance that grants the personal right to exercise freedom of conscience and religion, but I deny the legitimacy of syncretistic religion, which holds that all religions are equally true, equally false, and equally worthy of acceptance. Honest differences of understanding among Christian believers is one thing; putting Christian faith on a par with other world religions is something else again.

If Christianity could accommodate a syncretistic approach, the first-century church could have placed a statue of Jesus of Nazareth into the Pantheon at Rome. But that was never the goal of the apostles and early Christians. To the contrary, they advocated the distinctiveness of Jesus as Lord of all. Whether Jew or Greek, citizen or slave, powerful or weak—all people were pointed to Jesus as the one and only hope for eternal life. In the words of Paul:

> For even if there are so-called gods, whether in heaven or on earth (as indeed there are many "gods" and many "lords"), yet for us there is but one God, the Father, from whom all things came and for whom we live; and there is but one Lord, Jesus Christ, through whom all things came and through whom we live. (1 Cor. 8:5–6)

From the perspective of both Old and New Testament religion, it should be clear why the *first-in-sequence* commandment is also the *first-in-priority* commandment. The God who has called us out of bondage and saved us by a mighty work of redemption will not have a peripheral role in our lives. He will not serve as an occasional troubleshooter to bail us out of trouble in a crisis only to be banished to the twilight zone of our consciousness when things are going well. His claims are bold and exclusive. He will be everything to us, or he will be nothing. He neither seeks nor will he accept a position short of sovereignty in our lives.

> Honest differences of understanding among Christian believers is one thing; putting Christian faith on a par with other world religions is something else again.

When claims like those of the previous paragraph are made, Christians meet resistance. We are sometimes judged to be narrow-minded and intolerant. In a society where tolerance has become syncretism for many, the restrictions of "no other gods before me" and "no other name by which we must be saved" are offensive. In the words of Darrell W. Johnson:

> As long as we Christians say that Jesus is one of many saviors, we are warmly welcomed at the religious smorgasbord. We are welcomed even if we say that Jesus is the greatest of all the candidates for savior. But once we muster up the courage to say with Peter that Jesus is the *only* savior the world has, we are asked to leave the table.

The demand of exclusive allegiance within the Judeo-Christian tradition arises from two things. First, there is the matter of identity. Second, there are the unique deeds of God.

Divine Identity

Israel's call to a covenant relationship with deity began with these words: "I am the LORD your God." Quite literally, this preamble to the Decalogue begins: "I am YHWH your God." Standard English translations of Scripture render the tetragrammaton (YHWH) as "LORD." There is debate over how to pronounce the word, for pious Jews of later generations refused to pronounce the tetragrammaton lest they profane that holy name and violate the third commandment. Although some offer *Jehovah,* there is general scholarly agreement that *Yahweh* is the older and preferred pronunciation.

Yahweh, or Lord, is the covenant name of the God of Israel. Its first appearance in Scripture is in Exodus 3:13–15 when God appeared to Moses at the burning bush. Although the name had likely been used before that day, it henceforth had a special significance to the Israelites. The name means "I am being that I am being." The very name suggests that it would be inappropriate to speak of God as "was" or "will be"; his active being and eternal presence are expressed by a name appropriate only to the one who is from everlasting to everlasting and above all others. In response to his question at the burning bush (What shall I tell Israel about who sent me to be their deliverer?), Moses received this answer: "This is what you are to say to the Israelites: 'I AM has sent me to you.'" "Yahweh" or "I AM" signifies the God who is self-sufficient, unchanging, and faithful to his word.

In the New Testament, Jesus identified himself with this covenant name and role. In a confrontation with some enemies who had accused him of being "a Samaritan and demon-possessed," he countered with the claim that he was the Son of God and that "Abraham rejoiced at the thought of seeing my day." The response was an incredulous, "You are not yet fifty years old, and you have seen Abraham!"

> "I tell you the truth," Jesus answered, "before Abraham was born, I am!" At this, they picked up stones to stone him, but Jesus hid himself, slipping away from the temple grounds. (John 8:58–59)

There is no mistaking the double-edged claim here. Jesus both affirmed a continuous existence that included Abraham's day and claimed a title of Israel's deity for himself. Jesus' use of "I am" certainly connoted an identification with Yahweh to the people hearing him that day: they were ready to stone him for blasphemy. He could have put an end to their outrage by saying, "Oh, no! You misunderstood my meaning!" But Jesus allowed his statement to stand.

Scripture clearly declares that Jesus is one with the God of the Old Testament and that he is the eternal God come in flesh.

> In the beginning was the Word, and the Word was with God, and the Word was God. . . . The Word became flesh and lived for a while among us. (John 1:1, 14)

> Jesus Christ is the same yesterday and today and forever. (Heb. 13:8)

> Therefore God exalted him to the highest place and gave him the name that is above every name, that at the name of Jesus every knee should bow, in heaven and on earth and under the earth, and every tongue confess that Jesus Christ is Lord, to the glory of God the Father. (Phil. 2:9–11)

Divine Activity

God deserves first place in our lives not only because he is God but because of what he has done in history and in our lives. He is redeemer, deliverer, and savior. He is the one who "brought [Israel] out of Egypt, out of the land of slavery" (Exod. 20:2), and Jesus is the one "through whom we have now received reconciliation" (Rom. 5:11).

> To understand who he is and what he has done makes his demand both understandable and appropriate.

All religions acknowledge that humanity suffers from some form of bondage. Most offer deliverance through either some form of special enlightenment or a series of steps to liberation and new life. How different is the theme of biblical religion! Neither ancient Israel nor today's church is asked to free itself from bondage through secret knowledge or heroic performance. To the contrary, God does for us what we are totally unable to do for ourselves. The work of preaching the gospel is never performed faithfully by listing and binding a series of steps to liberation but by proclaiming freedom through divine activity that has already been performed on our behalf (cf. Luke 4:18–21).

Jesus faced and defeated the powers of sin and death. He understood the sources of our bondage as no one else ever had. So he acted in mercy and power to redeem us. Now he has the right to claim our exclusive and unshared allegiance. That is precisely what he does claim, and he will not accept anything short of that. But to understand *who he is* and *what he has done* makes that demand both understandable and appropriate. To quote Darrell Johnson again:

> He said, "Follow *me,*" while others said follow the law, follow the way of love or follow the Eightfold Path to Enlightenment. Jesus said, "Follow *me.*" Mohammed never made himself the issue of Islam. Buddha never made himself the issue of Buddhism. In fact, Buddha told his disciples that he could do nothing for them—they had to find their own way to enlightenment. A Jewish rabbi once observed that "no Moslem ever sings, 'Mohammed, lover of my soul,' nor does any Jew say of Moses, the Teacher, 'I need thee every hour,'" Jesus made *himself* the issue of his teachings—"Follow *me*—Abide in *me.*"

WHAT IS REQUIRED OF US

With God as center and circumference of one's life, the term *discipleship* has meaning. Yet the very word seems to have lost its serious content for most of us. We tend to assume that anyone who follows Christ is therefore a disciple. At a practical level, then, discipleship means such things as baptism, church membership, and the like. But that isn't nearly enough if we judge the call to discipleship by the standards Jesus urged on people during his personal ministry.

Jesus was followed by scores, hundreds, and thousands at various points during his earthly ministry. Still he kept calling for something more than mere following. Notwithstanding the fact that they had been baptized and were publicly identified with Jesus by trailing him around, he made it clear that more was required. He wanted the curious hangers-on who had found something meaningful in his messages to imitate his unreserved commitment to the kingdom of God. He asked for nothing less than the surrender of their total beings to righteousness. If we hear him in our own time, the challenge remains unchanged.

Our generation has produced millions of religious consumers but precious few people with a comprehensive devotion to Jesus Christ. These religious consumers read religious books but mistreat friends and family, listen to Christian music but don't approach giving ten percent of their income to the church, attend church expecting to be encouraged and helped but have no idea of what it would mean for them to abound in the work of the Lord. They feel free to criticize and church-hop without ever doing anything to build up a church.

A private religious life on a Christian's "own time" is not discipleship.

This approach to Christianity reflects a "cheap grace" mentality. Yes, salvation is altogether a work of grace. But the grace that cost God his Son is not cheap. Unreserved commitment in whole-life surrender to God is the only response worthy of someone who understands and accepts divine grace. This lifestyle of complete surrender to God reflects gratitude for grace, not an effort to win heaven or earn salvation.

A genuine disciple is one who follows Jesus' example of *total-life obedience* to God. Of course no disciple will ever be complete and flawless in her or his obedience to the divine will, but a real disciple sees that every element of life is now Christ's. Total-life obedience insists that one's whole life is dedicated to knowing and doing the will of God in every thought, every decision, every action. A private religious life on a Christian's "own time" is not discipleship. Only the conscious offering of one's total life with all its responsibilities, relationships, and resources will qualify as true discipleship.

A disciple who has "no other gods" dies to self daily and continually becomes more Christlike in everything. That person doesn't necessarily become a missionary to some third-world country, but he does bear faithful witness to Jesus Christ in everything he does. If he is a businessman, his "bottom line" is not profit but the nature of his business, its effects on environment, culture, and employees, and its role in defining his relationship with God. If she is a surgeon, her priorities put frightened people above tight schedules and compassionate truth-telling above convenient falsehoods. A Christian teenager puts Christ above the cultural idols of popularity, chemicals, or immorality.

CONCLUSION

The experience of the One True God requires that everything be submitted to his rule. Whoever we are, all our relationships, every responsibility, the totality of our possessions—everything must be surrendered to his sovereign claim to our allegiance. He must be Lord of all or not at all. He desires and demands to be center and circumference of our lives.

This commandment stands at the head of the list. How one reacts to it fixes the mind-set for receiving or rejecting all that follows. It forces each of us to settle the matter of priorities for living. Until the issue of this commandment is decided, nothing else about life can be in clear focus.

QUESTIONS FOR ADDITIONAL REFLECTION

1. How do you attempt to make God in your own image?
2. How do you approach the subject of your faith with unbelievers?
3. Does your faith "overflow in everything you do"? Why or why not?
4. Have you encountered any New Age ideas this week? How do you react to things such as healing crystals, reincarnation, and the like?
5. On what grounds do you accept Jesus' claim to be the only way to God?
6. How do you balance tolerance and love for people of other religions with the need to share God's truth and love with them?
7. Do you try to put God around the edges of your life rather than at the center? How does that affect your relationship with him?
8. Are there certain areas in your life you are more or less likely to involve God in? What are they? Why does this happen?
9. What has God done in your life that reminds you that he deserves your complete loyalty and obedience?
10. How does your relationship to God affect your finances? Your career? Your family? Your friends? Your church?
11. What matters more to you than anything else?

You shall not make for yourself an idol. . . . You shall not bow down to them or worship them.

Exodus 20:4–5a

CHAPTER FOUR

FROM THE SUBLIME TO THE TRIVIAL

2

"You shall not make for yourself an idol."

As water naturally tends to flow downhill, so does religion. Its inexorable movement in history seems clearly to be from exalted to degenerate, from holy to monstrous, from sublime to trivial. The second commandment is intended to stave off such an unworthy fate.

In the previous chapter we saw that the first commandment is a call to discipleship. It demands that we repudiate false gods and give our wholehearted allegiance to the One True God. We cannot straddle the fence but must declare our devotion to God. The second commandment goes a step further to warn us against worshiping the One True God under some false form or methodology.

As an illustration of what is at stake in this commandment, recall the experience of Israel while Moses was on the mountain receiving the Decalogue. The encamped nation came to Aaron and said, "Come, make us gods [or, perhaps better, a god] who will go before us" (Exod. 32:1). Moses' brother accommodated the people by taking gold from them and casting it in the form of a calf. The people reacted with the proclamation: "These are your gods, O Israel, who brought you up out of Egypt" (Exod. 32:4).

The second commandment goes a step further to warn us against worshiping the One True God under some false form or methodology.

While this sounds at first like a violation of the first commandment about "other" deities, closer examination shows that is not the case. As the people were celebrating the golden calf at its unveiling, Aaron stepped forward to act as priest for the people and said, "Tomorrow there will be a festival to the LORD" (Exod. 32:5). Because Aaron used the covenant name of Israel's God (LORD = Heb. YHWH), it is clear that he was not offering the calf as an alternate deity to Yahweh. The calf was meant to be a tangible representation of Israel's God. The people wanted something they could locate, see, and touch. They wanted something convenient, practical, and manageable. They wanted the transcendent, mystical, and incomprehensible reduced to a neat package. Aaron caved in to the demand and made them a mundane idol.

The challenge of this chapter is to understand and confess how idolatrous we mortals are. Its goal is to move us to a higher, nobler vision of God than provincial faith can envision. If we can ever succeed in tearing down the idols we have built to supplant God, life itself will be elevated to a higher plane.

IDOLATRY REDUCES GOD TO THE DEFINABLE

Israel Reduced God to an Idol

About six weeks had passed from the time Moses had climbed the mountain to receive the law from the Lord (cf. Exod. 24:15–18). The people waiting for him were accustomed to responding to someone they could see. Once it had been the Egyptian overlords who drove them to their daily labor. Lately it had been Moses. Their enslavement had created an unhealthy dependence on a visible leader. With Moses out of view for a month and a half, they were struggling with a powerful sense of insecurity.

With neither a shrine for worship (the tabernacle would come later) nor a leader in sight, the people went to Aaron and asked for a god. His response can be seen as an attempt to discourage the project. He told the people they would have to give their most valuable and prized possessions in order to have an idol. "Take off the gold earrings that your wives, your sons and your daughters are wearing," he demanded, "and bring them to me" (Exod. 32:2). Perhaps to his surprise, "the people took off their earrings and brought them to Aaron" (Exod. 32:3). If he had doubted the measure of their determination, this reaction showed he was mistaken.

With a dismal exhibition of personal weakness, Aaron gave in to the people and did as they had requested. On that disgraceful day, Israel reduced the glory of God to the image of a calf. (We should not be surprised it was a calf that was fashioned. Several Old Testament scholars have documented the fact that the calf or bull image was widespread as an object of veneration in the Ancient Near East. The Egyptian deity Amon-Re, for example, was represented as a bull. Later in Hebrew history, Jeroboam would set up calves at Bethel and Dan [1 Kings 12:28].) By its manufacture, the people were evidently inviting Yahweh to permit his glory and presence to be marked by that image. It was an unholy call to which he would respond with judgment. He ordered Moses to go down from the mountain and confront the people with his anger.

> Worshiping God in the form of a calf reduced the incomparable God to things known, defined, and customary.

These people were trying to make God visible. More than that, they were trying to "turn the tables" on the God who had created them in his own image by recreating him in the image of things they knew. This would make the unpredictable God predictable, the uncontrollable God controllable. It would reduce the incomparable God to things known, defined, and customary.

How Religion Reduces God

When religion reduces the incomprehensible and surprising God of Abraham to something defined and controlled by humans, mark it down that religion has become perverse. God can neither be reduced to his creation nor manipulated by it. But that is precisely what religion has tried to do over the centuries. We have tried to reduce him to a set of doctrines, make him the parochial deity of a certain denomination, or limit him to the narrow insights of a given tradition.

What religionists have failed to grasp over the millennia is that God is too big for us to comprehend, limit, or use to our purposes. Any attempt to represent him in a form such as a bull or other material entity is both preposterous and misleading. God must be worshiped as he is, not as we would like him to be. Faith must be placed in him, not in some magical icon.

Sacred Objects and Symbols

Human superstition is always directly involved in the making of idols. Some sort of "sacred object" is fashioned and assigned mystical powers. Whether it is a tiny calf or golden cross used as a good-luck charm, such superstitious use of icons is unworthy of reasonable people and degrading to the true meaning of spiritual life.

Please don't miss the point here. Religious art is not evil. After the episode with the golden calf, Moses would appoint a contingent of artisans to make the furniture and vessels to be used in the tabernacle. Employed properly to evoke a sense of awe and reverence before the Lord, ancient and modern art is compelling. It is only when these objects of art begin to be used as objects of superstition—as the ark of the covenant (cf. 1 Sam. 4:3) and brass serpent (cf. 2 Kings 18:4) came to be used among the Israelites—that they are evil.

As the most common symbol of Christianity, the cross has been used in both appropriate and inappropriate ways in the history of the church. Although some have barred the cross and all other symbols from the church, that is an extreme stance. Those of us who employ it in architecture and art must be on guard against fetishism (belief in magical charms), and we must remember that it is not the cross symbol that has authentic power in human life, but the reality to which it points.

Churches, Creeds, and Rules

More frequently in Christian tradition, it is not the worship of art that is our sin but the worship of theology, sect, or leader. In the recent past we have seen the emergence of evangelist "superstars" who have created little empires for themselves. They were willing to accept status for themselves that made their lifestyles resemble that of a petty monarch rather than the one adopted by a certain Galilean peasant.

Strange as it may sound, the human race has managed to trivialize God through churches, creeds, and moral exhortations. Am I saying that religion can get in the way of knowing Jesus? Exactly!

Religious legalism is itself a form of idolatry. It puts a list of right doctrines and required behaviors in the place of knowing God. It makes some church leader the judge of others' faith. It makes loyalty to the group or leader the test of acceptance with Christ. It reduces God to the definable.

You probably know people who believe that card playing is of the devil or that mowing your lawn on Sunday is a sin. There are people—very decent and serious people—who define spirituality in terms of abstinence from dancing, coffee, short skirts, and a variety of similar "vices." Many of us who grew up in very conservative churches know this mind-set from experience.

There was only one "right view" on issues ranging from having a glass of wine with dinner to attending movies to church architecture. And each of these "hot issues" was presented with as much zeal and dogmatism as the deity of Christ or the importance of the Lord's Supper.

Religious legalism puts a list of right doctrines and required behaviors in the place of knowing God.

In the meanwhile, these same churches said practically nothing about civil rights or materialism or world hunger. Did you ever wonder how that could have happened? A sociologist at Gordon College, Christian Smith, has advanced an interesting thesis to explain it:

> The reason is because, when it comes to the relatively important things in life (basic values and behavior concerning wealth, power, prestige, justice, security, peace, work, time, and so on), most Christians are indistinguishable from the world. Still, Christians know that they should be different from the world *in some way*—otherwise, what would Christianity mean at all? So, in an effort to establish some kind of Christian distinctiveness, attention and concern is focused on the trivial (which, by its very nature, does not require us to make difficult changes in our lives).
>
> In the end, it is okay to be entirely captive to the idols of mass-consumerism as long as we don't watch R-rated movies; perfectly acceptable to spend our entire lives pursuing a cozy, suburban affluence as long as we don't mow our lawn on Sundays; just fine to live a life completely indifferent to systemic, mass-starvation around the world as long as we don't drink beer.

> We, like the Pharisees, "strain out a gnat and swallow a camel" (Matt. 23:24).

As my friend who shared Smith's essay with me wrote in its margin, "Ouch!" Legalism makes issues of petty things to divert attention from its fundamental failure to grasp the gospel, to pursue the kingdom of God, and to demonstrate an authentic Christian lifestyle to the world. It allows people to create one of those located, defined, and controlled idols that takes the place of the Living God. Idols, after all, may take the form of carefully worked out arguments and ecclesiastical formulas as well as likenesses of animals or men.

Our human theological systems are not photographs of heavenly reality but flawed attempts to grasp holy things by means of the hints earthly things can provide. We must not confuse commitment to our particular theological perspectives with devotion to God. Our confused and unbalanced devotion to our theologies has divided us into different warring camps called "denominations" and has reduced us to partisan rivalry. The person who loves party more than truth is guilty of idolatry.

If we desire to take God seriously and move beyond our tendency to reduce the sublime to the trivial, we must stop majoring in nit-picked nuances.

> For the kingdom of God is not a matter of eating and drinking, but of righteousness, peace and joy in the Holy Spirit, because anyone who serves Christ in this way is pleasing to God and approved by men. (Rom. 14:17–18)

IDOLATRY DESTROYS MORALITY

When people cannot rise above their image of God, idolatry turns them away from holiness. When religion slides from the sublime to the trivial, the first thing to go is moral restraint. Paul wrote of this in the New Testament:

> For although they knew God, they neither glorified him as God nor gave thanks to him, but their thinking became futile and their foolish hearts were darkened. Although they claimed to be wise, they became fools and exchanged the glory of the immortal God for images made to look like mortal man and birds and animals and reptiles.
>
> Therefore God gave them over in the sinful desires of their hearts to sexual impurity for the degrading of their bodies with one another. They exchanged the truth of God for a lie, and worshiped and served created things rather than the Creator—who is forever praised. (Rom. 1:21–25)

It is inevitable that the worship of "created things rather than the Creator" will show itself in depraved behavior. Although he would later specify a variety of wicked things such as slander, murder, and greed, Paul named "sexual impurity" as the first and most direct consequence of idolatry.

When religion slides from the sublime to the trivial, the first thing to go is moral restraint.

The episode of the golden calf follows Paul's script faithfully. On the day of the festival that Aaron announced, the people "sacrificed burnt offerings and presented fellowship offerings. Afterward they sat down to eat and drink and got up to indulge in revelry" (Exod. 32:6). The Hebrew word translated "revelry" refers to sex-play (cf. Gen. 26:8). This sort of uninhibited and risqué partying was typical of the pagan religions of antiquity. Strange as it sounds to many of us, these drunken orgies were not considered immoral in those religions, but worshipful. Through God's holy eyes, however, they were viewed as corrupt and intolerable.

Pagan religion typically elevated sex to the realm of the divine. According to the pagan worldview, the mystery of fertility symbolized hidden, divine powers. The worship of the gods and goddesses of those religions was therefore sexual in content and rites. While the biblical view of things affirms sexuality and holds it in high regard, it sees God disclosing his unique divine powers in singular events of significance. Thus the Exodus and the Cross stand as nonrecurring events. It is these one-time acts, rather than the cyclical events involving fertility, that show us the nature of God. The worship rites of those religions have no status in the worship of Yahweh.

It has been affirmed that the three gods of our time are money, sex, and power. This observation simply reflects what people have always turned to when they turn away from worshiping and serving the True God: they seek meaning for their lives in the created things of God's world. They trivialize the Creator and fall prey to the seduction of created things. When we begin to wag our heads in disbelief at the greed, immorality, and exploitation of our world, we would do well to recall the biblical explanation: it is the result of idolatry.

There can be no genuine or lasting moral reform in our world apart from biblical faith. God cannot be represented in visible form, but his voice has been heard. The Word of God gives direction as to right and wrong, acceptable and unacceptable. The motivation for hearing and heeding that word is respect for God himself and for the image of God in other human beings. God's image is not in bulls, crystals, or medallions. It is in males and females of the human race. And the perfect specimen of the divine image is in Jesus Christ. A personal relationship with him is the single most important thing in human life.

IDOLATRY PROVOKES GOD'S JEALOUSY

The commandment against idols grows out of the jealousy of Yahweh. "I, the LORD your God, am a jealous God." Yahweh's name is "Jealous," we are told in Exodus 34:14. God's jealousy is not the peevish jealousy of a selfish and self-seeking deity. It is an even nobler jealousy than the jealous love of a husband or wife who is unwilling to share a beloved mate with a flirt.

God is not jealous *of* his people but *for* them. He longs to bless, not punish. Yet idolatry is such a terrible sin that it carries within itself the seeds of divine wrath—even to the third and fourth generations. That is, the sins that characteristically follow idolatry (e.g., greed, murder, disobedience to parents, faithlessness, etc.; cf. Rom. 1:28 ff.) defeat God's zeal to bless and elevate his covenant people. His anxiety to bless "to a thousand generations" is thwarted by sins that short-circuit all that is holy and ennobling in human experience.

In both Hebrew and Greek, the word for jealousy refers to single-minded devotion to an object. Thus the word itself is neither a virtue nor a vice. The object of the devotion determines whether jealousy is good or bad. If the object is self, the outcome is envy and hatred toward others. If the object is some evil end, a variety of sinful actions required to bring it about will be entailed. But if the object of the single-mindedness is a noble end, the word becomes altogether positive in tone. Unfortunately, our English word almost always has negative overtones.

God's jealousy for his covenant people is his consuming pursuit of their good. He seeks to honor his name among them. He wants to accomplish good things for them. This is the obvious meaning of the term in texts such as these: "Proclaim this word: This is what the LORD Almighty says: 'I am very jealous for Jerusalem and Zion, but I am very angry with the nations that feel secure'" (Zech. 1:14–15), and "I am jealous for you with a godly jealousy" (2 Cor. 11:2a).

CONCLUSION

Certain tribesmen in the Congo are said to regard one particular idol as their spiritual father. Revered by the people, the image is kept concealed in a deep pit. Missionaries to this primitive culture found that the people were afraid to draw it to the surface, for, they said, "If we look on the face of our father, we will die!" What a contrast to our situation as Christians. Our Father has revealed himself through the Son, so that Jesus could say, "Anyone who has seen me has seen the Father" (John 14:9b). God does not want us to cower before him in the way that superstitious people cringe before their totems and icons.

As Jesus told the Samaritan woman beside Jacob's well, the time has now arrived for God to be known by his true nature. He is not to be known through human, animal, or monster forms. He is to be known, instead, at a spiritual level, for the sake of his work in the world. As we know him through Christ, his mode of acting is not through mystical ritual, charmed icon, or holy place. He works through the direct union of Holy Spirit and human spirit in the arena of truth. "God is spirit, and his worshipers must worship in spirit and in truth" (John 4:24).

QUESTIONS FOR ADDITIONAL REFLECTION

1. Do you ever find yourself trying to put God into a neat package you can define and manage? Why do we do this?

2. What was at the root of the Israelites' insecurity while Moses was on the mountain? Do you struggle with insecurity? Is it for the same or different reasons?

3. How do you try to limit and control God? What borders and boundaries have you most commonly put on him?

4. How likely are you to make an idol out of the cross? Out of a religious practice? A leader?

5. Have you ever confused love for your particular church with love for God? How are they the same? How are they different?

6. How can you know when something becomes an idol in your life?

7. Do you think Christian Smith's analysis of Christianity cited in this chapter is fair or accurate? Why or why not?

8. Identify some areas of your life in which you "strain out the gnat and swallow the camel."

9. How do you react to the idea of God's jealousy for you?

You shall not misuse the name of the LORD *your God, for the* LORD *will not hold anyone guiltless who misuses his name.*

Exodus 20:7

CHAPTER FIVE

THERE'S SOMETHING ABOUT THAT NAME

3

"You shall not misuse the name of the LORD your God."

In the Lord's Prayer, Jesus reaffirmed the importance of this third commandment. He taught his disciples to pray: "Our Father in heaven, hallowed be your name" (Matt. 6:9). Against the American dictum that holds "There's nothing in a name," the Bible teaches there is something about the divine name that makes it sacred. Its misuse is a sin that will not go unnoticed by heaven.

Over the centuries, ancient Israelites attached such reverence to the covenant name of their God that they refused to pronounce it even in the public reading of Scripture. When coming to the name Yahweh, the reader would substitute the word *Adonai* (Lord) lest he "misuse" the holy name. This practice reminds me of the insistence in the '60s by some Christians that one should use only the pronouns "Thee" and "Thou" when addressing God. Is this commandment really about using a particular set of pronouns for prayer language? Is it about the intonation of God's name?

There is something about the divine name that makes it sacred. Its misuse is a sin that will not go unnoticed by heaven.

Reverence for the name of God does not preclude pronouncing the tetragrammaton (YHWH) or require a special set of pronouns in prayer. Things much more substantive are at stake here. What, then, does this commandment mean? Our responsibility in this chapter is to discover the significance of honoring the name of God and to identify some of the things that would constitute a misuse of it.

WHAT'S IN A NAME?

Names were far more significant in ancient times than in our own. Although many children were surely given names simply because of family tradition or because the parents thought the names "pretty," there is good evidence that many were named for some unique circumstance or in an effort to dedicate the child to God. One thinks of such children as Cain (possession, Gen. 4:1), Moses (draw out, Exod. 2:10), the children of Hosea (Hos. 1:3–9), Isaiah (May Yahweh save!), Daniel (God is my judge), and Timothy (God-fearer).

Even more revealing are the occasions where someone's name was *changed*, either by God or men, to signify something special about the character or role of that individual. Thus Abram (exalted father) became Abraham (father of many nations), Jacob (he grasps the heel) became Israel (he struggles with God), and Ben-Oni (son of my trouble) became Benjamin (son of my right hand). One also thinks of such nicknames as Boanerges (sons of thunder, for James and John, Mark 3:17) or Barnabas (son of encouragement, for Joseph, Acts 4:36).

God's Name Reveals His Essence

All this helps us understand the sacredness of the divine name and the seriousness of its misuse. *The name of God stands for the person he has revealed himself to be.* Since his name conveys something of his character, any use of it that does not show reverence is an affront to him. His name is to be "hallowed," honored as holy. The praise and honor of God must undergird everything his people do: "Ascribe to the LORD the glory due his name; worship the LORD in the splendor of his holiness" (Ps. 29:2). "Sing the glory of his name; make his praise glorious!" (Ps. 66:2). "Ascribe to the LORD the glory due his name" (Ps. 96:8a). "Not to us, O LORD, not to us but to your name be the glory, because of your love and faithfulness" (Ps. 115:1).

Although the patriarchs of Israel knew God by various *titles* (cf. Gen. 14:22; 16:13, et al.), biblical revelation focuses on the divine *name.* It was in connection with the Exodus that "Yahweh" was first used, not as another title, but as the personal name of Israel's God. What we know from the New Testament as the Holy Trinity was known collectively in the Old Testament under the mysterious name Yahweh. The character and works of God were both revealed and confirmed in the mighty redemptive acts that delivered the Hebrew nation from bondage in Egypt.

Jesus Shares God's Name

Israel's God, first known by titles and later by name, was ultimately and finally revealed in the person and work of Immanuel (Jesus) (cf. Matt. 1:23). Although the name—whether Yahweh or Jesus—does not confer power in any magical sense (cf. Acts 19:31), those who know that name are protected by it. "The name of the LORD is a strong tower; the righteous run to it and are safe" (Prov. 18:10). "Holy Father, protect them by the power of your name—the name you gave me—so that they may be one as we are one" (John 17:11b).

The apostle John locates the human experience of God and his redemptive work in the event of believing "in the name of God's one and only Son" (John 3:18; cf. 1 John 3:23). As a part of the faith process, baptism is peculiarly associated with "the name," either that of the Holy Trinity (Matt. 28:19) or of Jesus Christ (Acts 2:38).

Israel's God, first known by titles and later by name, was ultimately and finally revealed in the person and work of Immanuel.

Paul wrote of the glorification Jesus received at the conclusion of his earthly ministry by referring to the exalted name (Lord) he now bears:

> Therefore God exalted him to the highest place and gave him the name that is above every name, that at the name of Jesus every knee should bow, in heaven and on earth and under the earth, and every tongue confess that Jesus Christ is Lord, to the glory of God the Father. (Phil. 2:9–11)

The divine name is therefore a theological shorthand for all that is known of God and his deeds, how he has revealed himself to his creatures, and how we are enabled to share his fellowship. The name summarizes and stands for everything God is and has done. There is no wonder, then, that the misuse of that name is sinful and forbidden.

ABUSING THE HOLY NAME

To "misuse" ("take in vain" KJV) the divine name is literally to empty it or reduce it to nothingness. It is broad language designed to cover a wide range of behaviors. Since God has revealed himself to us as fully as we are able to receive divine revelation, we must take care never to show disrespect to him, his presence, his work, or his fellowship with his people. The God who is "I AM" will not allow his name to be used trivially and dishonorably without punishing those who dare to do so.

Because of the seriousness of misusing God's name—whether as Yahweh, Jesus, or any other form—it is essential that we name and explore the behaviors that would empty the divine name of its appropriate glory.

Perjury

It seems that in its original context the third commandment was intended to forbid what we generally term perjury. The ultimate pledge of truthfulness in a theocentric culture is to swear by the name of God. It was not forbidden for a Jew to swear by the name of God, but it was certainly a profane and vain use of the divine name to swear to a falsehood by it. "Do not swear falsely by my name and so profane the name of your God. I am the LORD" (Lev. 19:12). As Alan Cole has pointed out:

> A deeper reason for the prohibition may be seen in the fact that God is the one living reality to Israel. That is why His name is involved in oaths, usually in the formula 'as surely as YHWH lives' (2 Sam. 2:27). To use such a phrase, and then to fail to perform the oath, is to call into question the reality of God's very existence.

This helps one understand why false swearing is a misuse (emptying, reduction to nothingness) of the divine name.

Although some interpreters take the words of Jesus at Matthew 5:33–37 to be a prohibition of all swearing (oath-taking), such a view does not square with either Jesus' example or the larger body of New Testament information. Jesus responded to Caiaphas "under oath by the living God" (Matt. 26:63–64), and Paul swore by the name of God various times in his epistles (2 Cor. 1:23; Gal. 1:20; Phil. 1:8).

Jesus' teaching in the Sermon on the Mount is more correctly understood as a caution about invoking the name of God to take oaths in trivial matters. With their deceitful theology and ethical evasiveness, some people of Jesus' time made oaths indiscriminately, considering only those taken in the name of God to be binding. Jesus counseled against taking oaths trivially and instead urged an integrity that would allow one's "Yes" or "No" to be undoubted and without need of an oath for its certification.

Swearing to the truthfulness of one's testimony in legal documents or court proceedings is not a misuse of the name of God; giving false testimony in such a solemn proceeding is, however, a profane use of God's name. Neither is it improper to make vows to the Lord concerning one's spiritual life and service, but all such vows must be taken seriously and executed faithfully (cf. Deut. 23:21–23).

Profanity

This commandment is also a warning against profanity in ordinary speech. To use the name of God as many do today is certainly treating that holy name lightly. Blurting out some name or title of God as an exclamation of surprise, anger, or simply for the lack of another word is a serious misuse of his name.

The name of God is not "hallowed" when it becomes a convenient way to spew venom against or invoke a curse upon someone. Such language empties God's name of its meaning and insults his character and works as revealed in Scripture. Is there a more vicious prayer that can be prayed than "God damn you"? God is in the saving business and does not wish for anyone to perish (2 Pet. 3:9). To use his name to invoke an opposite fate on anyone dishonors him, his actions, and his motives.

An angry man was using God's name freely as he vented his anger at a clerk in a department store. Almost every sentence contained a request for God to consign someone or something to perdition. Standing with the enraged man was his eleven-year-old son who seemed unsurprised at such language. He was apparently accustomed to it. An older clerk walked over and asked, "Pardon me, sir, but do you always do your praying in public? And so loudly?"

"Praying!" exclaimed the man with still another oath. "What are you talking about?"

"Whether you mean to or not," said the soft-spoken, white-haired man, "you've been uttering one blasphemous prayer after another, asking the Lord to destroy everything you don't like. My God is not in the damning business, and you are giving this young boy the wrong idea about God: you are implying that God desires to condemn rather than to seek and save the lost."

By that point, of course, practically everyone in the store was listening. With blushing apologies, the customer left. His misuse of God's name had been exposed for what it was—terrible blasphemy and a complete misrepresentation of the nature of God.

Pretense

All forms of pretense in the name of God are censured by the third commandment. To use God's name to cover up an evil heart or to make oneself appear to be something one is not is therefore a violation.

A popular religious author and speaker admitted in a newspaper interview that many of the stories he has told over the years were untrue. For example, he had spoken often of playing professional baseball for the St. Louis Cardinals and of the time in World War II combat when his best friend died in his arms. Both were fabrications. How can someone consider it all right to lie in order to make a theological or moral point? Isn't that something like robbing a bank to fund a homeless shelter?

Jesus linked the larger issue of religious sham with misuse of his name in Matthew 7:21–23. "Lord, Lord, did we not prophesy in your name, and in your name drive out demons and perform many miracles?" some will ask him on the last day. But he will reject them because their use of his name was not coupled with genuine obedience. As William Barclay wrote: "Faith without practice is a contradiction in terms, and love without obedience is an impossibility." Invoking the holy name without pursuing a holy life is mere pretense; some of the harshest words of Scripture are reserved for such persons (cf. Matt. 23:1 ff.).

Presumption

This commandment also warns against a presumptuous use of the name of God. Making a long list of the things that have been done in the name of God would make us sick. The crusades, inquisitions, slavery, South African apartheid—all were done in the name of God.

Many fund-raising schemes used in religion surely belong under this heading. One TV preacher mailed 122,000 pieces of brown paper to people on his mailing list. He called each a "resurrection prayer rug" and suggested that health, prosperity, and miracles went with it—for those who sent it back with a "seed faith" check for $10 or more. Another went on the air and pleaded for $4.5 million from his viewers to keep God from "calling him home" by the end of the month. The absurdity of portraying God as a hostage-taker is a flagrant misuse of the divine name.

From foul-mouthed pagan to fund-raising preacher, the possibilities of emptying God's name of its honor and power seem endless. In contrast to such a spirit, there is an attitude toward God that the Bible calls "the fear of the Lord."

HONORING THE NAME OF GOD

Scripture describes the spirit that hallows God's name as the *fear* of the Lord. This spirit is at once an attitude of esteem and awe before the majesty of God and a confidence in his mercy and love. While Yahweh has revealed himself as a mighty and terrible God who is to be feared, he does not invoke the cringing, groveling terror that worshipers of pagan gods felt.

The people of God's covenant community respect him. When he speaks, the people listen; when he commands, they obey; when he is disobeyed, he does not hesitate to punish. There is thus a stability about his relationship with his worshipers that was never present in any of the pagan myths. Their gods were petty, unpredictable, and untrustworthy. But Yahweh is the same yesterday, today, and forever.

When God reveals himself, his powerful presence so overwhelms his people that they often react in fear. That is when he says, "Fear not" (Gen. 15:1; Judg. 6:23, et al.). His movements toward his people are always designed to bless, never to terrorize. It is precisely because of this that the fear of God is a holy attitude of awe, reverence, and gratitude.

Scripture describes the spirit that hallows God's name as the *fear* of the Lord.

The famous *Shema* calls Israel to love God with heart, soul, and strength (Deut. 6:5). In light of the third commandment, though, it is interesting to note that the text continues with this appeal: "Fear the LORD your God, serve him only and take your oaths in his name" (Deut. 6:13).

In the New Testament, fear remains a proper motivation for serving God. Thus we are commanded to "purify ourselves from everything that contaminates body and spirit, perfecting holiness out of reverence (Gk. *phobos* = fear) for God" (2 Cor. 7:1). Husbands and wives are to learn mutual submission "out of reverence for Christ" (Eph. 5:21). And Peter gave this broad exhortation: "Show proper respect to everyone: Love the brotherhood of believers, fear God, honor the king" (1 Pet. 2:17).

Indeed, the New Testament also knows the type of fear that is simply terror and anxiety; but Christ has liberated us from bondage to the "fear of death" (Heb. 2:15) and taught us of a perfect love that "drives out fear, because fear has to do with punishment" (1 John 4:18).

A classic text on the fear of God as a holy motivation is Psalm 111.

> Great are the works of the LORD; they are pondered by all who delight in them. Glorious and majestic are his deeds, and his righteousness endures forever. He has caused his wonders to be remembered; the LORD is gracious and compassionate. . . . He provided redemption for his people; he ordained his covenant forever—holy and awesome is his name. (2–9)

> The fear of the LORD is the beginning of wisdom; all who follow his precepts have good understanding. To him belongs eternal praise. (10)

In light of what the Bible teaches about the fear of God, it is imperative that we hallow the name, person, and works of God. Both in creation and in redemption, he is greatly to be feared. Our fear is not the paralyzing terror one might feel before a hot-tempered judge; it is the honor and respect due God because of who he is and what he does.

Old ways of thinking and behaving cannot be broken by formulas, but they will give way to reverence.

Indeed, fearing him is the beginning of all wisdom. As was observed in chapter 1, all that is holy must be rooted in reverence. Understanding how to live righteously and happily in this world is impossible until we see God and fear him. While legalism offers its methods and formulas for solving life's problems, the Bible says the fear of the Lord is the foundation. Old ways of thinking and behaving cannot be broken by formulas, but they will give way to reverence. "Through the fear of the LORD," wrote Solomon, "a man avoids evil" (Prov. 16:6b).

CONCLUSION

Perjury, profanity, pretense, and presumption are affronts to the name above all names. Beyond these obvious and gross irreverences, Christians are called to exalt and cherish all holy things. But when we, as the body of Christ, allow ourselves to be distracted from holiness, we offer the world an irreverent view of God and his work. Division, pettiness, and hostility in the church dishonor the name of the one who purchased it with his blood.

We show that we do not fear our Holy God when sacred matters lose their importance to us—as when we turn the Lord's Supper into a ritual or reduce heaven-and-hell themes to tasteless jokes. Things that are treated seriously in Scripture deserve to be taken seriously by people who fear the name of the Lord.

And we certainly do not fear God when we excuse our personal sins. Cheating husbands and wives simply do not fear God. Dishonest business dealings, neglect of the homeless, mistreatment of children—all reflect a lack of regard for God and the image of God borne by the people in our world.

Would that more of us could be described as God-fearing men and women. Would that we not only use the word "hallow" in prayer but that we actually hallow his name in all we do—for there really is something in a name.

QUESTIONS FOR ADDITIONAL REFLECTION

1. Would God prefer us to have a special, pious reverence for his name in worship or to revere his name by holy living?
2. How does the name of the Lord protect those who know it?
3. Have you ever taken an oath or vow in the name of God? If so, how serious were you about that oath or vow?
4. What do you think of the older clerk's reaction to the angry man's profanity? How could you react in that situation to show respect for the name of God?
5. How do you think people are affected when they hear God's name used repeatedly in profane ways

at work, at school, on TV, and in other public settings?

6. Do you know situations where God's name is invoked to further evil purposes? If so, what kind of situations?
7. Has God's revelation ever overwhelmed you to the point of fear? What was that like?
8. How is "fearing the Lord" different from the fear of punishment?
9. How does the fear of God lead to wisdom?
10. Does your fear of God lead you to treat sacred matters with the importance they deserve?

Remember the Sabbath day by keeping it holy. Six days you shall labor and do all your work, but the seventh day is a Sabbath to the LORD *your God.*

Exodus 20:8–9a

CHAPTER SIX

MY TIME IS HIS TIME

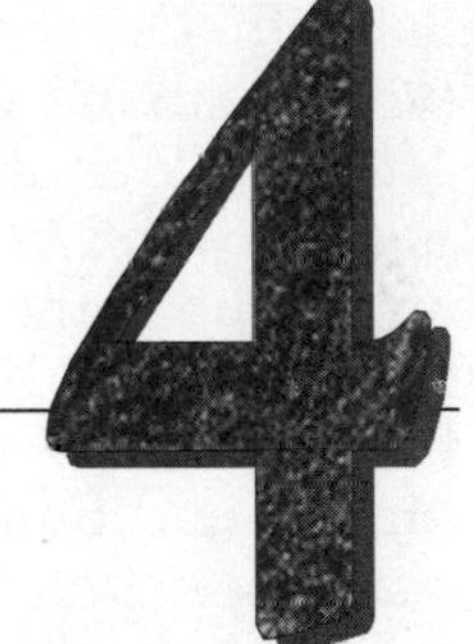

"Remember the Sabbath day by keeping it holy."

The fourth commandment is the first of the only two commandments given in positive rather than negative form. It enjoins a rhythm of rest and work, with one day from each week observed as a day holy to God. Hardly any other commandment in the Decalogue is given as much emphasis in Mosaic legislation as this one; its violation carried the death penalty (Exod. 31:14; cf. Num. 15:32–36).

Throughout the Old Testament, Sabbath law was integral to the life of Israel as God's covenant people. Even in the year's busiest times of plowing and harvesting, the Sabbath was to be kept faithfully (Exod. 34:21). Preexilic prophets such as Isaiah taught the people to view the day not as a burden but as a delight (Isa. 58:13), and postexilic prophets like Nehemiah emphasized it strongly as part of the spiritual renewal God sought among the people (Neh. 10:31; 13:15–22).

In the New Testament, we discover that the Sabbath was at the center of several controversies in the life of Jesus. We read of Jesus attending the synagogue on the Sabbath "as was his custom" (Luke 4:16), yet there are at least six recorded confrontations between him and his contemporaries about appropriate behavior on the Sabbath. Did it violate the Law of Moses to pluck grain while walking through a field on the Sabbath? (Mark 2:23–26). Was it sinful to heal a man with a withered hand (Matt. 12:1–8), a crippled woman (Luke 13:10–17), an invalid at the Pool of Bethesda (John 5:1 ff.), or a man who had been blind from birth (John 9:1 ff.) on the Sabbath? Or were these actions merely violations of rabbinical tradition? Jesus raised this question for debate among "experts in the law" in Luke 14:1–6 and proceeded to heal a sick man in their presence.

Today, the Sabbath question remains at the heart of several theological and practical differences among believers. Seventh-Day Adventists insist that observance of the Sabbath is still God's will and that the general Christian shift from Saturday to Sunday as the church's primary day of public worship is unjustified. Among those who affirm the first day of the week as the principal day of corporate worship for the church, there is dispute as to whether it should be called "the Christian Sabbath" and/or regulated by the Old Testament strictures about permissible and forbidden activities on that day.

There is also a legitimate scholarly dispute as to whether the Decalogue *initiated* Sabbath observance or merely *formalized* it for Israel. If it was merely a formalization and the people had been accustomed to the Sabbath as a day of rest, why did Moses give such detailed instructions in Exodus 16:22 and the verses following? Why would he need to explain the requirements of "a holy Sabbath to the LORD" with explicit particulars about gathering, baking, and boiling if the institution was already established? On the other hand, if the command initiated a *new* practice, Genesis 2:3 is a bit confusing: "And God blessed the seventh day and made it holy, because on it he rested from all the work of creating that he had done." God had deemed that day as holy long before the Law was given. But perhaps this is merely an instance of *prolepsis*, where two distant events are joined together as if they happened simultaneously (cf. Gen. 3:20; Matt. 10:4). Certainly there are plausible arguments on each side; there is no way to settle this debate with certainty.

What we do know about the Sabbath is that the commandment was subject to abuse among the Israelites. By the time of Jesus, it had clearly become a heavy-handed and oppressive requirement rather than a delightful and positive aspect of their religion. The legalistic traditions added to the Sabbath law by its interpreters were part of what Peter dubbed "a yoke that neither we nor our fathers have been able to bear" (Acts 15:10b).

In this chapter, we will explore the original meaning of the fourth commandment for Israel, consider the enlightening teachings of Jesus regarding the Sabbath institution, and trace out some of the enduring value of the Sabbath command for Christians.

THE MEANING OF THE SABBATH

The Sabbath, as such, is a distinctively Jewish observance. It was a special ordinance between Yahweh and

Israel, a "lasting covenant" and a "sign between [God] and the Israelites forever" (Exod. 31:16–17).

The Hebrew noun translated "sabbath" means cessation or rest. It is derived from a verb meaning to cease, to pause. As a day of rest and worship, the Sabbath was to be observed on the seventh day of the week, Saturday. In its full form, the Sabbath commandment reads as follows:

> Remember the Sabbath day by keeping it holy. Six days you shall labor and do all your work, but the seventh day is a Sabbath to the LORD your God. On it you shall not do any work, neither you, nor your son or daughter, nor your manservant or maidservant, nor your animals, nor the alien within your gates. For in six days the LORD made the heavens and the earth, the sea, and all that is in them, but he rested on the seventh day. Therefore the LORD blessed the Sabbath day and made it holy. (Exod. 20:8–11; cf. Deut. 5:12–15)

This expanded form of the command highlights at least three things. *First,* it requires work as well as rest and affirms what was earlier in this chapter called a "rhythm" between the two. Both are holy before our God. *Second,* the command to cease from routine work on the Sabbath applied to slaves, foreigners, and animals as well as members of the covenant community of Israel. *Third,* the precedent for rest on the seventh day is found in the Genesis account of creation, in which God created the world in six days and rested on the seventh.

As Wilfred Stott has pointed out in an article on the Sabbath in *The New International Dictionary of New Testament Theology:*

> The day then was looked on as a cessation from labour, a pause, a rest, but this with a view to its being dedicated to God, an opportunity for getting to know God and for worshipping him.

Devotion to God

The fundamental principle embodied in this commandment is that *mankind needs a fixed time of spiritual devotion to God,* and that requires a day of rest from ordinary affairs. Work itself is a good and even holy thing, but its physical and mental stress can destroy men and women. One day per week is needed for recuperation from the "grind" we have created in our hectic culture. Yet this is not to say that the Sabbath principle is merely pragmatic in that it lets us "recharge our batteries" so we can get back to work and be more productive. The day is meant to find its primary employment not in entertainment or selfish indulgence but in devotion to the worship and service of God.

The day is meant to find its primary employment not in entertainment or selfish indulgence but in devotion to the worship and service of God.

During the Old Testament era, Saturday (the seventh day) was a holy day of rest. Individuals and families were expected to plan their week with that day in view. Advance preparation was made for such things as meals and fires in order to avoid having to tend to them on the Sabbath. Lighting a new fire, for example, was not permitted after sundown on Friday and before sundown Saturday (Exod. 35:3).

Not Intended to Prohibit Necessary Functions

Although most of us know the Sabbath law through what it prohibited, we need to understand that the Law of Moses permitted such necessary work as priestly functions, caring for the sick, and saving the life of an animal. Jesus cited these generally understood "exceptions" to the rule of total inactivity during a dispute with the Pharisees, who challenged his right to pluck grain (Matt. 12:1 ff.): "Your disciples are doing what is unlawful on the Sabbath," said his challengers. But using the example of David, Jesus replied that the Law of Moses does not prohibit eating to sustain life. Furthermore, Jesus used irony to rebuke his critics by reminding them that "on the Sabbath the priests in the temple desecrate the day and yet are innocent." Of course the priests did not "desecrate" the Sabbath by performing their duties on that holy day and neither did anyone else—including Jesus and his disciples. No one desecrates the Sabbath by performing necessary functions such as eating, required tasks of worship, or humanitarian deeds of kindness or lifesaving.

As the debate continued, he asked "If any of you has a sheep and it falls into a pit on the Sabbath, will you not take hold of it and lift it out?" Again, his point was to deny that the fourth commandment was ever intended to be taken to the extremes to which the rabbis had gone in their interpretations of it. So he made his final point with these words: "How much more valuable is a man than a sheep! Therefore it is lawful to do good on the Sabbath." In a word, the Sabbath commandment was something very different than Jewish tradition had made it. It was a much gentler and more humane ordinance than they had appreciated. What had happened to the Sabbath requirement over the centuries?

Legalistic Misinterpretation

In the period between the testaments (400 B.C. until the time of Jesus), Judaism came to be distinguished under two types. In Israel proper and in Mesopotamia, a rigid and legalistic approach to the Law of Moses evolved. Among the Jews of the diaspora (Jews living in predominantly Gentile countries), a more liberal and often compromised form of interpretation arose. The legalistic interpreters were determined to preserve all the commandments in their most literal forms. Thus they even began the practice of building a "hedge" around each commandment. That is, they set out to give detailed lists of things that were involved in keeping each commandment. Within their intention was the prohibition of even those things that might lead one into the danger of disobedience.

The *Mishnah* (the body of Jewish oral law that was written down by the end of the second Christian century) devotes the first tractate of its second division to the Sabbath issue. "Forty save one" actions are listed that were prohibited on that day. Among these are such deeds as separating two threads, writing as many as two letters of the alphabet, tying a knot, carrying something from one place to another, etc. Each of the prohibitions in turn generated debate as to what constituted an offense of its type. Did wearing an artificial limb constitute a violation of the injunction against carrying an item from place to place? Some rabbis said it did, but others disagreed. Could a tailor take his needles home on Sabbath eve? Could a scribe carry his pen home Friday afternoon? The issues of controversy were endless.

Intended to Bless

The Law of Moses was never intended to make the will of God so burdensome. Thus Jesus made this general statement about Sabbath observance: "The Sabbath was made for man, not man for the Sabbath" (Mark 2:27). Legalism turned a beautiful and pleasant day into a harsh and hateful ritual. It made the day a burden among its adherents and an object of ridicule to observers. From the start, God had intended for the day to be a blessing rather than a burden to his covenant community. Families and friends could be together, devotion to God could be shared with other believers, and the spirit and the body could be refreshed. But legalism always forgets the ideal of law in its pursuit of trivia.

SATURDAY OR SUNDAY? SAME OR DIFFERENT?

Although some people speak of Sunday as the "Christian Sabbath," the term is an oxymoron and never occurs in Scripture. The Sabbath belongs to Israel as an ordinance, and Christ's church has never been bound to its observance or subject to judgment concerning it.

Sometimes it is claimed that the church took the Sabbath idea from Judaism and gradually changed its day of worship from the seventh day of the week to the first. A look at the New Testament evidence shows nothing of a gradual transition from one day to the other. Sunday, the first day of the week, has been the special day of worship for the Christian church from the day of its founding (Acts 2:1). Sunday is the day on which Christ rose from the dead (Matt. 28:1). It was on a Sunday that the Holy Spirit came upon the apostles and founded the church (Acts 2:1 ff.). New Testament literature presents Sunday as the day of the church's worship (cf. Acts 20:7; 1 Cor. 16:2). Early on, in fact, Christians began referring to Sunday as "the Lord's Day" (Rev. 1:10; cf. *Didache* 14.1). While Sunday did not become a state holiday in the Roman Empire until Constantine made it such in 321, it has been the significant day of Christian worship from the church's founding day on Pentecost of A.D. 30. Having said all this, however, the real meaning of the Sabbath is not concerned with the primary days of weekly worship under the two covenants. The principle underlying the Sabbath rule is relevant for all people in every generation.

THE ENDURING PRINCIPLE OF THE SABBATH

To what degree is Christian behavior on the Lord's Day to be governed by Sabbath regulations? Rather than trying to translate all the nomadic-agrarian rules of the Old Testament into our world—and falling into the trap of legalism—it is wiser to look for the undergirding principle of this commandment and then apply it to our life situations.

Surely it is an extreme to say that a family cannot pick up a basket of food and carry it to the park for a Sunday picnic because of the Sabbath rule against carrying objects. On the other hand, however, it is an equally mistaken extreme to hold that Christians may treat Sunday as just another business-as-usual day. After all, it is the *Lord's* Day and should be used accordingly.

Sunday ought to be used in ways that indicate our devotion to God. It is a day for public worship with the people of God. It is a wonderful time for an otherwise busy family to be together and to strengthen its ties of communication and love. It is probably the best day in the week for seeking out and being with someone who is sick, struggling in his or her spiritual life, or unsaved. These are things that may be difficult to do on ordinary workdays of the week, and they seem especially appropriate as ways to honor the Lord on *his* day.

Much of the fruitless haggling over the relationship between the Sabbath and the Lord's Day trace to a fundamental oversight as to the purpose behind the fourth commandment. While the Sabbath commandment has no exact equivalent in the New Testament, its underlying principle is relevant to all people at all times in history.

Our Time Belongs to God

The critical truth embodied in the fourth commandment may be summarized this way: *Our time is really God's time, and we must be faithful stewards in how we use life.*

The first three commands have called us to honor God by (1) putting him first in our *devotion* (no god other than the True One); (2) sanctifying him in our *hearts* (worshiping him faithfully); and (3) honoring him with our *lips* (respecting his holy name). The fourth commandment calls for us to glorify God by our use of priceless *time.* Whatever years we have on Planet Earth are God's gift to us and are to be used for his purposes. The old hymn expresses this principle with these words: "Take my moments and my days; let them flow in ceaseless praise."

Time is the very essence of life, and the Bible contains several emphatic reminders of our obligation to use it wisely: "Teach us to number our days aright, that we may gain a heart of wisdom" (Ps. 90:12). "Be very careful, then, how you live—not as unwise but as wise, making the most of every opportunity, because the days are evil" (Eph. 5:15–16). "Make the most of every opportunity" (Col. 4:5b).

When time is wasted, it cannot be replaced; and when it is misused, it cannot be refunded for wiser handling.

Christian teachers appear to have done a better job of teaching stewardship of money and talent than of time. Yet time is the one absolutely indispensable item in this list. Lost money can be replaced by effort and thrift, squandered talent can be reclaimed and put to use, but time is irreversible. It moves relentlessly in only one direction, and the only part of it you control is the present moment. What is wasted cannot be replaced, and what is misused cannot be refunded for wiser handling. It is Satan who leads us to misuse time, and it is a spiritual victory to learn to use time well.

Good stewardship of time under the Lord Jesus Christ involves learning to live a well-ordered life with appropriately allotted time for family, friends, exercise, rest, work, recreation, and sleep as well as for prayer, Bible reading, worship assemblies, and Christian service. We disgrace ourselves and dishonor God when we live in such a frenzy that we alienate people, break health and sanity, or neglect our spiritual lives. Good religion is, among other things, good sense about the apportionment of precious time.

Many books have been written in the past few years about time management. Perhaps reading one would be helpful for you. But read with a particular perspective. Don't read with a view toward answering the question, What is the best way for me to use time so as to make money? but read with the view, What is the best way to use time to the glory of God?

Stephen Covey's best-selling *Seven Habits of Highly Effective People* has an excellent section on time management. His summary of everything that is important on the subject is reduced to only five words: "Organize and execute around priorities."

The stewardship of your life under God involves giving priority to your family. Don't let a busy life crowd out your husband, wife, or children. Don't let your family go to pieces simply because you don't arrange your time to be with the people you love most in all the world. After all, the people God has put closest to you in human experience constitute a sacred trust from him. Families that fail don't set out to self-destruct. Often the members of a given family simply allow their lives to get so fragmented by the careless use of time that they have no time to get to know each other, understand each other, or love each other.

Build time into your life for making and cultivating friendships. Set aside time to do things you enjoy—whether reading, painting, music, long walks, or whatever—things that rest and refresh your soul. Don't abuse your body, but realize that it is a temple of the Spirit of God. Everything about you and your life can be to God's glory if you use your time well. "So whether you eat or drink or whatever you do, do it all for the glory of God" (1 Cor. 10:31).

The Right Balance

A Time for Work

"Six days you shall labor and do all your work" (Exod. 20:9). Apparently there are some people who fail to see that a full work week is envisioned in the fourth commandment. The desire to do less and less while receiving more money and leisure time for it is a blight on the modern world and a character defect within the person.

The best interest of human beings is served by work. In the Garden of Eden, prior to the Fall and curse, humans were given the responsibility of working. "The LORD God took the man and put him in the Garden of Eden to work it and take care of it" (Gen. 2:15). Scripture demands honest labor of all who are able to work. "For even when we were with you, we gave you this rule: 'If a man will not work, he shall not eat' " (2 Thess. 3:10).

Work is honorable, and no person whose life is committed to God's glory resents it or envies the person who somehow manages to get along without it.

A Time for Rest

Though humans are meant to work, God did not create our bodies and minds for constant tension and uninterrupted exertion. There has to be a time of backing away for rest and renewal. "The seventh day is a Sabbath to the LORD your God. On it you shall not do any work" (Exod. 20:10).

Most of us know the term "workaholic." A workaholic isn't simply someone who works hard or puts in long hours. He or she is the person whose identity is so caught up in *doing* that there is no time for simply *being*.

A workaholic is so identified with a job or role that he has no identity apart from performing it. Eugene Peterson is probably correct in pointing to this as a spiritual defect and giving this counsel as a corrective: "At regular intervals we all need to quit *our* work and contemplate *his,* quit talking to each other and listen to him."

Rest is as honorable as the honest labor that makes it seem so sweet.

After you work hard and complete your task, don't feel guilty for enjoying a period of rest and relaxation. Rest is as honorable as the honest labor that makes it seem so sweet. The two go together in God's plan for a healthy lifestyle.

A Time for Worship

Christians worship God in many settings, both private and public. But Sunday is a time for heightened sensitivity to spiritual concerns. Worship simply must not be taken lightly by someone who believes that his or her time belongs to God (cf. Heb. 10:25).

Work, rest, worship—these constitute the elements of *balance* that all believers need to incorporate into their lives. Each has its critical place in imitating, enjoying, and praising God. No one may neglect any one of them without harming the purpose God has for his or her total life.

CONCLUSION

Have you ever heard someone, perhaps with a stark tone of belligerence, say, "It's my life, and I'll do with it what I want"? Maybe you've even said it yourself in a moment of exasperation. But surely all of us know better.

In my heart of hearts, I know that my life is not mine to use according to some selfish purpose. I have been bought by the blood of Christ. A ransom price has been paid to set me free from Satan's clutches. I belong to God. So my first responsibility is to order my daily life so that it honors divine ownership. Following his counsel, I must live with the right balance of work, rest, and worship. After all, my time is his time.

QUESTIONS FOR ADDITIONAL REFLECTION

1. What caused the Israelites to turn a positive commandment into what this chapter calls "a heavy-handed and oppressive requirement"?
2. Have Christians ever turned a gift of God into something oppressive and burdensome? If so, what? How? Why?
3. Do you feel a personal need to set aside time from ordinary life affairs to focus on God? If so, what changes would you need to make in your schedule?
4. In what areas of spiritual life have modern Christians created lists of *can*s and *can't*s that cause endless—and perhaps pointless—controversy?
5. How do you spend a typical Sunday?

6. Compare your stewardship of time to your stewardship of money. With which are you more careful? Why?

7. How do your prioritize your use of time? Do you do it consciously or simply "go with the flow" of life?

8. How do you divide your time among work, rest, and worship?

9. Ideally, how *should* you divide your time among work, rest, and worship? How much difference is there between this answer and your answer to the previous question? How can you decrease the difference?

Honor your father and your mother, so that you may live long in the land the LORD *your God is giving you.*

Exodus 20:12

CHAPTER SEVEN

GOD AMONG THE GENERATIONS

5

"Honor your father and your mother."

What do you value most about your family? What are your best memories of your mother and father? Are you one of the increasing number of people whose memories of home are tarnished by abuse or abandonment?

Everyone longs for the warmth and security of family. The ideal home provides warmth when the world is cold, safety when other places seem hostile, and light when the surroundings are dark. It offers love around the dinner table and laughter under a shared roof; it generates and nurtures faith as the family goes to church together. Family is mutual respect, forgiveness, and dreams.

Rudyard Kipling wrote this about family: "All of us are we—and everyone else is they." That line captures the essence of family for me. A family is a circle of people held together by the cement of love. Its members are uniquely loyal to each other. They nurture each other, stay alert to one another's needs, and see to it that no one in the group is ever excluded.

But all too frequently we hear horror stories about spouse abuse, child molestation, or mistreatment of elderly parents, and we wonder what has happened to the concept of familial love.

The biblical notion of "honor" within the family unit has been severely compromised. In this chapter, we will examine the principle of honor in connection with the fifth commandment of the Decalogue. The goal of the chapter is to help us reestablish honor for the elderly within our homes.

As practically every student of the Ten Commandments has pointed out, the fifth commandment is a *transitional* command within the law. As John Durham put it:

> The transition from Yahweh's expectation of his people in relation to himself to his expectation of his people in relation to the human family is this commandment establishing a norm for the relationship with father and mother.

The first four commandments focus on Israel's relationship with God. The final six define the association of the covenant community with humankind. At the pivot point between the obligations of loving God and loving one's neighbor stands the commandment about family integrity.

Against the bleak future some sociologists see for the family, this commandment calls us to see its indispensable and proper place at the center of life.

THE MEANING OF THE FIFTH COMMANDMENT

Its Recipients

Contrary to the interpretation commonly given this commandment, its principal force is not as an admonition to young children and adolescents to follow their parents' orders. Adults are the ones who received the Decalogue at Mount Sinai, and our reading of this commandment must keep that in mind.

This is not meant to imply that infants and children are not within the scope of the Ten Commandments. Of course they are to respect and submit to their parents. This was the common understanding of every culture in the Ancient Near East. Both Old and New Testaments assume that parents have authority over their children. To think, however, that this assumption includes an unrestricted right to coerce children or to punish them harshly is simply wrong. To the contrary, Paul wrote: "Fathers, do not exasperate your children; instead, bring them up in the training and instruction of the Lord" (Eph. 6:4; cf. Col. 3:21).

The focus of attention for this commandment is the treatment of elderly parents by their adult children. This is apparent not only because of its original audience but also because of the controversy Jesus had with the Pharisees about the meaning of honoring parents (Matt. 15:3–9). The precise issue at stake in that dispute was leaving elderly parents destitute and thereby failing to obey the command about honoring father and mother. (We'll discuss this passage more in the coming pages.)

Its Emphasis

The verb *honor* means more than paying attention to someone's request. It carries the idea of elevating, esteeming, or giving special deference to someone. The second of only two positive Decalogue commands, the fifth commandment is a particular application of a general attitude of respect for older people that runs throughout the Hebrew Bible. "Rise in the presence of the aged, show respect for the elderly and revere your God. I am the LORD" (Lev. 19:32).

The Old Testament regards human parents as the channels of God's gift of life. God is to be reverenced as the source of all life, and parents are to be esteemed as participants with him in passing life to their children. Thus the Scripture reads: "Listen to your father, who gave you life, and do not despise your mother when she is old" (Prov. 23:22). Anyone who attacked or cursed either of their parents was to be put to death (Exod. 21:15, 17). It should be noted that in this legislation mothers are given equal status with fathers. Such a posture is unusual in the literature of the Ancient Near East but consistent in *biblical* statements about the family.

The Old Testament regards human parents as the channels of God's gift of life.

Its Promise

In the New Testament, Paul calls this commandment "the first commandment with a promise" (Eph. 6:2). Its explicit promise is that people who observe the requirement of the fifth commandment will "live long in the land the LORD your God is giving you." In light of the death penalty for anyone who abused his or her parents, it is not hard to find the primary meaning of those words. They are also probably intended to carry the secondary meaning—consistent with all the Old Testament says about the wisdom of elderly persons—that those who honor their parents will have a longer (and better) life than those who neglect their counsel.

Its Neglect

In a discussion with some Pharisees about their misproportionate emphasis on tradition over law, Jesus said:

> Why do you break the command of God for the sake of your tradition? For God said, "Honor your father and mother" and "Anyone who curses his father or mother must be put to death." But you say that if a man says to his father or mother, "Whatever help you might otherwise have received from me is a gift devoted to God," he is not to "honor his father" with it. Thus you nullify the word of God for the sake of your tradition. You hypocrites! Isaiah was right when he prophesied about you: "These people honor me with their lips, but their hearts are far from me. They worship me in vain; their teachings are but rules taught by men." (Matt. 15:3–9)

In the preceding scenario, adult children, moved by greed, shirked their responsibility to elderly parents. In an effort to skirt the requirement of the Law and still be held in regard within the community, they declared the money or goods that should have gone to support their parents to be *korban*—a gift devoted to God (cf. Lev. 27:9, 16). But Jesus delivered a stinging rebuke against their legalistic tricks that permitted them to set aside specific provisions of the Decalogue. Their grossly misplaced priorities were revealed in their efforts to sidestep the fifth commandment.

This case study points out that Jesus' interpretation of the fifth commandment put the responsibility for taking care of elderly parents on their children. While this clearly does not exhaust the meaning of "honor" to parents, it is fundamental.

Its Exceptions

There are times when children are discharged from this duty, but selfishness and greed can never be the basis of such a suspension of responsibility. When one's family stands in the way of faithfulness to the kingdom of God, family ties must be sacrificed for Jesus' sake (Matt. 10:37–39). Similarly, parents who have betrayed their trust to children by abandonment or abuse are hardly in a position to make manipulative claims against their children in the name of religious duty. Other factors may also be relevant.

THE HEART OF THE FIFTH COMMANDMENT

Seen in the context of modern values, this commandment highlights several important truths that our society ignores. It is important for believers to affirm what the larger culture tends to discount.

The Vital Role of Family

The home is the basic social unit, and no nation can remain strong whose families are unstable. It is older than and more formative to character than the church. Parents within the family unit stand, to use a legal expression, *in loco dei* (in the place of God) to their children. This means that their responsibility is not to be taken lightly. Being a mother or father is the most demanding and important role any of us will ever fill.

The Blessings of Showing Honor

The fifth commandment carries the connotation that children need parental love, guidance, and wisdom. Although the commandment focuses on the obligation of the children, we should not overlook the motivation that surely lies behind it. While it protects the status and rights of parents, its worth is more to the children who show honor than to the parents who receive it. Children who resist their parents forfeit a measure of civility, maturity, and spirituality. They also make it more difficult for themselves to respect others in authority, including their Father in heaven.

Children who resist their parents forfeit a measure of civility, maturity, and spirituality.

How to Show Honor

Parents who have loved and cared for their offspring deserve gratitude and care in return. Sometimes this means financial support, but more often it means showing little courtesies like phone calls, making time to visit, and providing emotional support. This commandment was given in a pre-Social Security world. It assumes a support of elderly parents that fewer people will be called upon to provide; but it envisions a subtler set of needs that can be overlooked because the more obvious ones are being met. Paul echoes the sentiment of this commandment by saying that people "should learn first of all to put their religion into practice by caring for their own family and so repaying their parents and grandparents, for this is pleasing to God" (1 Tim. 5:4).

The following case study, about a man I will call Arnold, supplies a living illustration of this point. After careful consideration, Arnold decided to place his father in a health-care facility. The decision was not made because of a desire to avoid taking care of his dad. It was a practical and wise decision in view of the health problems involved. His father understood the decision, even though he would have preferred to stay in the home he had maintained since his wife's death seven years before. But that simply wasn't possible under the circumstances. I have no reason to think that Arnold had to pay any of his father's bills or take financial responsibility for him. His father was secure enough under government and private insurance programs that he could meet all his own fiscal needs. For more than two years, though, I watched Arnold meet the subtler needs of his father. He visited him frequently. He helped him stay in touch with his family and friends. He took him to church when his father's health permitted. In every way he knew, Arnold showed his esteem and love for his father. Neither his dad nor those of us who knew him ever had the impression that Arnold "dumped him" at the nursing home in order to avoid being "bothered" with the old man.

Society's Need to Show Honor

This commandment should put all of us on notice about respect for older people in general. The treatment of a society's older members has varied greatly from culture to culture. Among the Chukchi Siberian tribe, it was once considered an oldest son's sacred duty to take his father's life when the latter's powers begán to wane. In times past, Eskimos exposed their old people to death by freezing. In opposition to such examples, the most honorable of all ancient traditions was that found among the Hebrew people. Instead of segregating people by age, the young honored the old and the old taught the young. Older people among the Israelites were kept alert and involved in the community because their counsel was constantly sought (cf. Job 12:12).

Generation to Generation

When Norman Rockwell was illustrating *Saturday Evening Post* magazine covers in the 1930s and '40s, he often depicted grandmas with gray hair fixed in a bun, dressed in gingham, mixing a batch of muffins. Grandpa was typically portrayed in slippers and a baggy sweater, dozing—rimless glasses askew—in a rocking chair. It was considered appropriate then for grandparents to stay home and bask in the sunset of life.

Grandparents today are anything but Normal Rockwell stereotypes. Today's grandmother may be taking an aerobics class, and granddad may be running a ten-kilometer race. While the images of typical activities may have changed, one thing has remained the same: grandparents still want to share time and experiences with the children of their children.

Showing honor among all the generations of a family is God's will. Blessings will flow in all directions when the commandment to do so is obeyed.

OUR PERSPECTIVE ON AGING

The family context is the place where issues of aging, intergenerational support, and death can be handled most constructively. The last thing most Americans want to think about, however, is their mortality. But I'm dying. And so are you. In spite of all our efforts, we will never stop the aging process or cheat death.

The family context is the place where issues of aging, intergenerational support, and death can be handled most constructively.

The average life span for women is about seventy-five years; men live to be about seventy-two. Human cells divide about fifty times and then start falling apart like old jalopies! "The length of our days is seventy years—or eighty, if we have the strength" (Ps. 90:10a).

As best science can figure it, there is a kind of built-in biological limit programmed into the cells of the human body. Laboratory experiments done with fibroblasts from a human embryo point to an outer limit for the life of our species. Even when those cells were grown under optimal conditions, death followed after fifty doublings. This means that the life span of humans will probably never be much greater than it is now in America.

Yet, we are bombarded with media images that make us hate our aging bodies, drive us to spend millions annually on surgery with no purpose except to make us look falsely younger, and deny older people the respect and deference most cultures give them. The department store cosmetic counter is not a fountain of youth. And most cultures would be baffled by American men dying their gray hair, for, in those cultures, it would be equivalent to forfeiting part of their masculinity and life.

Yes, the human body is worth preserving. Yes, we are stewards before God of life and health as well as money and talents. But we need to exercise caution in our pursuit of health and fitness. Philip Yancey put it this way:

> And yet, in the end, the health club stands as a pagan temple. Its members strive to preserve only one part of the person: the body, which is the least enduring part of all. . . . Physical training is of some value, Paul advised Timothy, but godliness has value for all things, holding promise for both the present life and the life to come (1 Tim. 4:8). As I pedaled, straining against computer-generated hills, I had to ask myself: What is my spiritual counterpart to the Chicago Health Club? And then, more troubling: How much time and energy do I devote to each?

Thoughts about our mortality need not be morbid, but we need to remember where our hope lies. It is not in this world, but in the world to come. It is not with the physical body, but with the resurrected one.

Soren Kierkegaard considered our awareness of death to be the central characteristic that distinguishes humans from animals. Martin Luther wrote:

> Even in the best of health we should have death always before our eyes [so that] we will not expect to remain on this earth forever, but will have one foot in the air, so to speak.

We need to take death into account lest we forget what God has done to defeat it. Death will not have the last word. Mortality will be swallowed up by life through the decisive triumph of Jesus Christ.

CONCLUSION

The fifth commandment probably makes more demands on people of our time than it did on the ancient Israelites. For one thing, more people are living longer than ever before. The advances of medical science have reduced infant mortality, curbed the devastation of childhood diseases, and brought adults through injuries and health crises that would have made them die much younger a hundred years ago. Just think of the contrast, for example, between the percentage of people who live to be seventy or older in the United States versus those in third-world countries. For the first time in history, getting old is commonplace rather than extraordinary.

In cultures where relatively few "survivors" reach their seventh decade and beyond, it is more natural to esteem and give deference to them. Our culture has many old people, and this fact alone may make honoring them more difficult.

The issue in this commandment is made more complex by virtue of the fact that older people have begun to be thought of as a threat to the rest of society. Aged citizens of the United States are a significant political power bloc. Young people resent having to pay higher taxes to fund the increasing pull on the Social Security system. Some social scientists have estimated that as much as 40 percent of the federal budget will be devoted to the care of the elderly by 2040. Unless our politicians become more responsible and creative in addressing the issue of public support for the elderly, we could move quickly into a time of hostility, rather than honor, toward older people.

Much of the current debate over euthanasia and assisted suicide is rooted in a whole society's attitude toward old people. If we continue to communicate the message that only those young enough to earn and contribute by their work are truly worthwhile to our culture, more older people will be stripped of their self-respect and thus of their ability to maintain the respect of others. Americans praise *doing* above *being*, whereas the Bible defines worth in terms of being (existence in God's image) rather than doing (talent and productivity). People who are merely tolerated, because they no longer work and produce surplus value in their culture, can easily feel that their only remaining obligation is to "die and get out of the way."

Much of the current debate over euthanasia and assisted suicide is rooted in a whole society's attitude toward old people.

Regardless of the success or failure of public policy toward our parents, grandparents, and great-grandparents, the biblical mandate for believers remains the same. Individuals, families, and churches must be unselfish with their respect and love for their elders. Honor among the generations is a critical factor—both in maintaining intergenerational civility and in preserving the dignity of our older citizens.

QUESTIONS FOR ADDITIONAL REFLECTION

1. How does honoring one's parents help make life longer or better for a person? How has honor for your parents contributed to your personal welfare?
2. Have you ever known of people using religion as an excuse for not meeting their family obligations? If so, how?
3. Honor is a two-way street. Has your relationship with your parents made it easy or difficult to honor them? If you have children, what sort of relationship are you creating with them?
4. "Being a mother or father is the most demanding and important role any of us will ever fill." Do you agree or disagree with this statement from this chapter? Explain.
5. How has your relationship with your parents affected your relationship with your heavenly Father?
6. Is it easier to meet the financial or emotional needs of your older relatives?
7. How do you honor older members of your family? of your work environment? of your church?
8. How can one honor a parent who has Alzheimer's disease?
9. Do you try to avoid the physical signs of aging? Why or why not?
10. Do you ever think about your own death? How does that thought make you feel?

11. How does the issue of respect for parents relate to the issues of euthanasia and physician-assisted suicide?

12. What creative possibilities for affirming older people and helping them preserve their dignity exist in your church? What additional ones might be worth exploring?

You shall not murder.

Exodus 20:13

CHAPTER EIGHT

THE VALUE OF A HUMAN LIFE

6

"You shall not murder."

It appears that we have created a culture that places very little value on human life. America now holds the dubious distinction of leading the industrialized world in violent crime and murder. The annual homicide total in the United States topped 20,000 in the mid-1970s. After a one-year drop, it grew to 23,040 in 1980 before declining for several years. The numbers began rising again in 1985, hitting 23,760 in 1992.

Periodic crime bills passed by state and federal legislatures can't contain brutality. Building more prisons doesn't seem to reduce the number of violent criminals. At some point we are going to have to acknowledge that politics cannot solve what is fundamentally a moral, cultural, and spiritual problem.

Proof that our culture has spawned a new form of violent crime that is particularly notable for its randomness and brutality is abundant.

A nineteen-year-old male in Washington, D.C., randomly shot into a nearby car while riding around in the city in 1992. He killed a thirty-six-year-old woman. "I felt like killing somebody," he explained. It was the third shooting the man had allegedly committed in the twenty-six days since his release from juvenile detention. He smiled for the cameras when he was arrested, refused to stand when he was convicted of murder, and clapped when his life sentence was announced.

The father of Michael Jordan was murdered in 1993 by two eighteen-year-olds who had staked out a roadside rest stop in North Carolina. They shot James Jordan, dumped his body, and drove away with his car. One of the young men was on parole after serving only two years of a six-year sentence for trying to kill a man by smashing his head with an ax. His accomplice was awaiting trial for hitting a sixty-one-year-old woman in the head with a cinder block during a robbery, fracturing her skull and causing a brain hemorrhage.

No story of violence has been more horrifying than a Houston double murder in 1993. Six young men, ranging in age from fourteen to eighteen, were arrested for the rapes and strangulations of two teenaged girls. "Hey, great!" one of them said after hearing they were being charged with murder, "We've hit the big time." Only one day before the murders, one of the other defendants had appeared on a local TV program about gangs. Hoisting a beer to the camera, he boasted, "Human life means nothing."

The courts' handling of the violence that is tearing our society apart astonishes and mystifies the public. For example, a violent attack on a seventy-two-year-old man in the course of a robbery left him near death. A transit policeman pursued the assailant, shooting him in the back and paralyzing him. The criminal sued, and a New York jury awarded him $4.3 million for his "pain and suffering." The victim of the crime got an extended stay in the hospital; the perpetrator got a cash award. Something is wrong with the system. Terribly wrong.

Violence, brutality, murder—they multiply in a culture that has no respect for the sanctity of human life.

THE COMMANDMENT IN CONTEXT

Contrary to the lack of respect for human life reflected by much of our society, the Bible consistently upholds the sanctity of life. It is in this context that the sixth commandment is framed. The sacredness of human life is grounded in the biblical truth that males and females are created in God's own image. On the sixth day of the creation week, God said, "Let us make man in our image, in our likeness" (Gen. 1:26a). The text continues: "So God created man in his own image, in the image of God he created him; male and female he created them" (Gen. 1:27).

Everything the Bible says about the worth and dignity of humanity is rooted in the creation story. Women and men are not accidental outcomes of purposeless natural events. All human beings are valuable because they were called into being to bear the glory of the God who willed them to exist.

Against the modern tendency to define the worth of an individual in terms of wealth, talent, or position, the Bible teaches that a single human being is of infinite intrinsic value (cf. Matt. 16:26). It is not your father's bank account or your cousin's expensive car or a celebrity's special talent that defines his or her importance. Being created in God's own likeness is what makes a person worthy of respect and fair treatment.

Also contextual to the sixth commandment is the time of Noah. As he and his family stepped out of the ark to become the new fountainheads of the human race, Yahweh called their attention to the sacredness of human life and stated the penalty that was to be exacted from anyone who might dare take a human life without justification. "Whoever sheds the blood of man [a Hebrew expression that refers to taking life], by man shall his blood be shed; for in the image of God has God made man" (Gen. 9:6). The regulation was clear and unequivocal that anyone who showed such irreverence toward God as to take innocent human life was to pay with his own. It was against this background that the Decalogue prohibited murder.

In an early section of the Sermon on the Mount, Jesus commented on several specific provisions of the Ten Commandments (Matt. 5:13–48). When the sixth commandment was raised for discussion (Matt. 5:21–26), he insisted that it was never intended merely to prohibit what we have come to think of as first-degree murder. It was intended, instead, to safeguard the sanctity of human life in general. Thus he taught that any form of anger, rage, or malice toward another human being puts one in jeopardy of judgment from God. These things not only can lead to murder but are wrong in themselves. Showing disdain for others by racist attitudes, sexist behavior, or any other form of contempt is evil in the eyes of God.

One of the final warnings in Scripture is that murderers will have to take their place "in the fiery lake of burning sulfur" (Rev. 21:8). This is not to say that murder is the unpardonable sin. To the contrary, even people who had participated in the murder of Jesus of Nazareth were offered forgiveness for their awful deed (Acts 2:36–38). But any person who has such callous disregard for human life as to commit murder and not repent of that act will suffer the eternal wrath of God that is called the "second death."

Showing disdain for others by racist attitudes, sexist behavior, or any other form of contempt is evil in the eyes of God.

ALL KILLING IS NOT MURDER

Some have offered an interpretation of this commandment that makes it an absolute prohibition of taking human life, regardless of the circumstances. In view of one of the passages already cited from Scripture in this chapter, it is clear that such an interpretation is not true.

There is a degree of ambiguity in the word *kill* that makes it less than the best translation for the word used in this commandment (e.g., "Thou shalt not kill" KJV). The word *kill,* which embraces all forms of life taking, has been replaced in most modern translations with the more precise word *murder.*

Does the sixth commandment prohibit all life taking, including self-defense or punishment? Clearly it does not, for the penalty for breaking it is death.

> Anyone who strikes a man and kills him shall surely be put to death. However, if he does not do it intentionally, but God lets it happen, he is to flee to a place I will

> designate. But if a man schemes and kills another man deliberately, take him away from my altar and put him to death. (Exod. 21:12–14; cf. Deut 19:11–13)

If the command in question is an unqualified prohibition of all life taking, it would have prohibited the Hebrew community from executing the stated penalty for its violation. Such a reading turns Scripture on its head and makes the Old Testament incoherent and self-contradictory.

All murder is killing, but not all killing is murder. The Law of Moses condemned all acts of murder (e.g., killing someone to steal his money), but it did not condemn all acts of killing (e.g., executing a thief-murderer).

The Old Testament distinguishes at least three types of homicide. First, there is *premeditated murder.* This is the evil act of hating, planning harm, lying in wait, and taking another's life. Or it may be the taking of someone's life in the course of committing some other crime against him, such as the case in the previous paragraph of taking someone's life while trying to rob him (cf. Num. 35:16–21). Second, there is *accidental homicide.* If, for example, two men are working together and one accidentally causes a rock or heavy machine to fall on the other, crush him, and kill him, no murderous act is involved. The Bible considers cases of accidental death and specifies the duty of the larger society to protect those who cause death without intending to do so. Such people could flee to one of six "cities of refuge" in Israel's territory and claim sanctuary (cf. Num. 35:6, 22–28). Third, there are cases of *self-defense* or *justifiable homicide.* "If a thief is caught breaking in and is struck so that he dies, the defender is not guilty of bloodshed" (Exod. 22:2).

Of these three types of homicide, then, only the first is envisioned by the sixth commandment. The implications of this truth are important for us to trace out.

SOME THINGS *NOT* FORBIDDEN

Among other things that may be implied by the previous discussion, we can be sure that capital punishment, police action, and justified war are not condemned by the biblical principle of respect for the value of human life.

Capital Punishment

Capital punishment is certainly not forbidden in Scripture. The Old Testament not only permitted but required the death penalty for crimes such as murder (Gen. 9:6), rape (Deut. 22:5), kidnapping (Exod. 21:16), and several other offenses that were affronts to Yahweh's theocratic rule of the nation (cf. Deut. 13:5; 17:2–7).

In the New Testament, the right of the state to enforce the death penalty is upheld consistently. Both testaments were produced by the same God, after all, a God whose character does not change. Both reveal him to be a God of love, but his love has never allowed him to ignore *justice.*

Jesus did not question the right of a government to take the lives of certain criminals. In a conversation with Pilate while on trial for his own life, he granted the right of Rome to execute criminals and protested only the false charges that had been made against him. In his own words, Pilate's authority to oversee capital punishment was given "from above" (i.e., by God). In similar circumstances, the apostle Paul took the same position (Acts 25:11).

The New Testament grants human government the right to regulate conduct within the state. With regard to criminal activity in particular, Paul wrote: "But if you do wrong, be afraid, for he does not bear the sword for nothing. He is God's servant, an agent of wrath to bring punishment on the wrongdoer" (Rom. 13:4).

In both testaments, the death penalty is the prerogative of the state and its agents, not private citizens. Neither Jews nor Christians are allowed under their Scriptures to bear personal malice or to "get even" for criminal offenses against them. No private citizen may take the law into his or her own hands with the approval of the Bible to become judge, jury, and executioner. But the same Bible that prohibits personal retaliation (Rom. 12:19) has ordained a legal system to handle these matters under law (cf. Rom. 13:1–5).

Rehabilitation and deterrence are never the central issues with regard to capital punishment in the Bible. The single issue is justice. Scripture makes a commonsense distinction between villain and victim; it condemns the one and defends the other. Modern societies make too little of the distinction that exists between these two classes of citizens.

Rehabilitation and deterrence are never the central issues with regard to capital punishment in the Bible. The single issue is justice.

No Christian could rejoice in the taking of a criminal's life in an electric chair, by lethal injection, or before a firing squad. The ideal situation would be to create a world where the necessity for punishing criminals would be eliminated. But in a nonideal society, punishment is necessary.

Police Action

Police action is not prohibited in Scripture. Exodus 32 relates the sad episode in Israel's history involving the worship of a golden calf at the base of Mount Sinai. When Moses came down from the mountain and saw what the people had done, he said, "Whoever is for the LORD, come to me" (Exod. 32:26b). In response to his challenge, the tribe of Levi gathered to stand with him. Then he gave these instructions: "This is what the LORD, the God of Israel, says: 'Each man strap a sword to his side. Go back and forth through the camp from one end to the other, each killing his brother and friend and neighbor' " (Exod. 32:27). In effect, he "swore in" the Levites to be a police force that would deal with an outbreak of idolatry in Israel's camp. That police force was given the right to execute people who were defying Yahweh's rule.

In the New Testament, Peter teaches that Christians must acknowledge the right of the state and its agents to punish criminals:

> Submit yourselves for the Lord's sake to every authority instituted among men: whether to the king, as the supreme authority, or to governors, who are sent by him to punish those who do wrong and to commend those who do right. (1 Pet. 2:13–14)

Justified War

Participation in a justified war is not prohibited by this commandment. The nation of people to whom this command was originally given fought both defensive and punitive wars with the blessing of God. Israel was hardly out of Egypt, for example, when the Amalekites attacked them at Rephidim. Moses called on Joshua to be the head of an army, to organize troops, and to fight against the attackers (Exod. 17:8–16). When the security of the young nation was at stake, Israel had a moral right to form an army and to seek the blessing of God in fighting against its enemies. Much later in the nation's history, King Saul was told to undertake a war of extermination against the Amalekites for their consistent history of aggression against Israel and their depravity of heart (1 Sam. 15:1–3). Israel fought such defensive and punitive wars not as a necessary evil or in defiance of the will of God; they fought them as the avenging sword of the Almighty.

In the New Testament, soldiers were not required to give up their careers in view of the coming of the Son of Man (cf. Luke 3:14; Acts 10). To the contrary, one should recall that Romans 13 says that the state exists under God's authority for the purpose of executing divine wrath against people who do evil.

Sometimes people have to support the use of deadly force not because they are pleased to see harm come to other human beings but because its use is the only way to show respect for those who have been harmed by criminals.

But what is a "justified war"? A war is morally justified when a nation uses its military force to turn back a genuine threat to the security of its people or to rescue others from harm. Just as self-defense is justified for an individual against an attacker or for a city's police force against a dangerous gang, so is a nation justified in defending itself against international murderers.

Again, the use of such deadly force as has been described above is not something that God-fearing people want to see happen. Ethical people employ such force only with an attitude of regret. But the question here is not preference but moral justification. Sometimes people find themselves in the awful situation of having to support the use of deadly force (e.g., sitting on a jury, paying taxes that purchase bombs, serving on a police force) not because they are pleased to see harm come to other human beings but because its use is the only way to show respect for those who have been harmed by criminals.

SOME THINGS FORBIDDEN

A number of contemporary social issues are, in fact, ethical issues that relate to the sixth commandment. It would be an unpardonable oversight not to raise them for consideration in this chapter. There are at least three that deserve to be mentioned.

Abortion

On January 22, 1973, abortion became a legal option for pregnant women in the Unites States of America. According to the Alan Guttmacher Institute, over twenty-eight million legal abortions were performed in the following twenty years. Approximately forty-three hundred abortions are performed every day in this country, one every twenty seconds. While it is true that the Bible nowhere says "You shall not abort," the sixth commandment has been understood by both Jews and Christians across the centuries to include the repudiation of abortion. Heirs to a profound respect for unborn and newly born human life and aware of Jesus' example of welcoming little children, many generations of Christians apparently never questioned a uniform antipathy toward abortion among believers. They made no argument for a woman's "right to choose" or for "individual conscience" to settle the matter and stood adamantly against abortion and infanticide.

There is good scientific reason to argue for conception as the decisive time of humanization. When the chromosomes of sperm and ovum unite, a new DNA complex is created. In other words, it is at the instant of conception that the new entity receives the genetic code that will forever set it apart as belonging to the human race. It is not church dogma or uninformed tradition that suggests conception by human parents as the criterion of human status but modern microbiology.

Furthermore, we take for granted the right to life of an infant in a mother's womb—except when debating abortion. Prenatal medicine allows the diagnosis of many fetal problems through such means as amniocentesis and ultrasound. Drugs have been administered to the unborn, blood transfusions have been given to fetuses, and surgery has been performed inside the womb. If we rejoice in these advances in prenatal medicine that *save* life, should we not deplore its use to *destroy* life?

Sacrificing one human life to save another (abortion to save a mother's life) is one thing, but disposing of a human life at will (abortion to avoid parental inconvenience) is something else again. According to statistics from Planned Parenthood, no more than 7 percent of abortions are primarily traceable to the "hard cases"—

mother's life or health (3 percent), baby's health (3 percent), or rape (1 percent). A decent and moral society must affirm the sanctity of human life. The permissive attitude toward abortion that prevails in America today is inconsistent with such an affirmation.

Suicide, Physician-Assisted Suicide, and Active Euthanasia

Derek Humphrey's suicide manual *Final Exit,* Jack Kevorkian's various "suicide machines," and the Hemlock Society's media campaign for the legalization of physician-assisted suicide have put these topics on the agenda for public debate. Or perhaps they have been forced into the national consciousness because of the poor way in which medicine, theology, and public sentiment have dealt with terminal illness and death. In either case, they cannot be avoided.

The term euthanasia means "good death." Passive euthanasia is the withholding or discontinuance of treatment for dying patients under certain conditions. Living wills, for example, allow people to indicate that they do not wish to be placed on respirators or subjected to "heroic measures" to resuscitate them as they are dying. Passive euthanasia permits death to occur when there is no reasonable hope of a person's recovery. Active euthanasia, however, is a very different matter. It is intervention designed to terminate life. It is frequently called "mercy killing." Both ethically and practically, this is a quantum leap from simply permitting the death of a hopelessly ill woman or man.

Active euthanasia and suicide are in direct conflict not only with the Decalogue but with the Hippocratic Oath. Our western heritage has taught us to affirm, nurture, and give aid to people who are sick, injured, and in pain; the antithesis of that heritage is to adopt a policy of destroying troublesome or traumatic life.

Recent swinging of the pendulum toward tolerance for suicide and euthanasia communicates the message that terminally ill people have a duty to get out of the way of the living. Suppose a cancer patient for whom treatment has been ineffective tells his or her family, "I know I'm a terrible burden to you, and I wonder if I shouldn't just take my own life!" I can imagine two different responses with very clear messages.

Passive euthanasia permits death to occur when there is no reasonable hope of a person's recovery. Active euthanasia, however, is a very different matter.

"What do you mean!" says one family. "You are critical to our lives. We love you, and you will never be a burden to us. Never!" That answer communicates a relationship within the group that inspires a will to live for the patient and affirms compassion and support by the others.

"Perhaps we should think about that," replies another family. "You might suffer toward the end, and we don't have enough money to hire nurses so you can be cared for while we are at work." With such openness to the idea of helping her die, what feelings would likely go through the mind of that patient?

No one comes onto Planet Earth with an exemption from suffering. Physician-assisted suicide or some other form of active euthanasia is neither the moral nor practical solution to pain. Companionship and support, loyalty and compassion, love and kindness—these are better answers to the problem of suffering than carbon monoxide or lethal injection. Our call is not to become executioners.

Self-Inflicted Harm

Respect for life also prohibits self-inflicted harm of the sort so many of us foster. The abuse of alcohol, drugs, and tobacco is not consistent with respect for one's life as a gift from God or her body as a temple of the Holy Spirit. And the gluttonous and obese person must ask himself how his lifestyle is fundamentally different from that of the drug abuser or smoker. Any deliberate abuse of our bodies is a reflection on our regard for God's wonderful gift of life to creatures in his own image.

There is a modern school of thought that denies the reality of free will and refuses to hold people accountable for their behaviors. But this viewpoint has fallen into disrepute as society has begun to realize that we cannot live with the consequences of classifying everyone a "helpless victim." In place of this self-defeating approach, any number of helpful groups modeled on Alcoholics Anonymous have based their approach to addictive behaviors on personal responsibility. And AA's Twelve Steps are founded on the biblical model of repentance and accountability.

CONCLUSION

A close look makes it apparent that the sixth commandment has a much broader application than one might have thought at first. It applies to more persons than contract killers. It touches on the world all of us must share.

Abortion, euthanasia, and self-abuse are issues that touch our lives daily. All of us have to deal with the personal matter of keeping our hearts free of the desire for revenge against people who hurt us. Prejudice toward people of a different race, national origin, or religion is still an unresolved problem.

None of these problems can be dealt with successfully until we learn the value of a single human life.

QUESTIONS FOR ADDITIONAL REFLECTION

1. What does it mean that males and females of the human race are "in the image of God"?

2. How do you define your worth? What about the worth of others?

3. If anger were a crime, could you be convicted? What about malice? Racism? Sexism?

4. Is capital punishment ever appropriate? Is it appropriate only for cases of first-degree murder?

5. Which wars do you classify as "justified wars"? World War II? Vietnam? The Persian Gulf War? The civil war in Yugoslavia? How do you distinguish them?

6. How do you believe Christians should respond to the issue of abortion? Should it be accepted? Opposed quietly? Protested peacefully? Fought with any and all available means?

7. What is your position on passive and active euthanasia? Do you see a meaningful distinction between the two?

8. Has anyone in your family ever faced a decision about euthanasia? How was it handled?

9. Are there ways in which you do not treat your body in an appropriate manner? How can you change those things?

10. Are there applications of this commandment that come to your mind that are not mentioned in this chapter?

You shall not commit adultery.

Exodus 20:14

CHAPTER NINE

KEEPING MARRIAGE INTACT

7

"You shall not commit adultery."

About a quarter of a century ago now, a book titled *Open Marriage* proposed a new form of marriage "contract." It opted for letting each pair write a contract based on mutual desires and preferences that would be recognized in law. Around the same time, a member of the Maryland Legislature introduced a bill to legalize a "renewable" three-year contract for marriage, while others opted to abandon the marriage concept altogether for cohabitation without legal ceremony or regulation.

The theory behind all these approaches seems to have been that mate selection, living together, and separation are purely private matters that ought to be free of public interference. Collectively they challenged the traditional concept of marriage as a lifelong relationship. They deemed the seventh commandment's prohibition of thoughtless trashing of marital commitments as no longer necessary to a liberated society.

The results of this pendulum swing toward liaisons without commitment and its concurrent devaluation of faithful monogamy were disastrous. The divorce rate in the United States reached an all-time high of 5.3 per 1,000 in 1979. The number of children living with only one parent stands at approximately eighteen million—26.7 percent of all children under age eighteen. Divorce on demand has proved to be a disaster for children, for their hurt and angry parents have no idea how to cope with either their own anxieties or those of their emotionally tender offspring. And divorce has a way of perpetuating itself into succeeding generations.

People are realizing that making commitments and keeping promises is at the heart of being authentic human beings.

In the 1990s, the pendulum seems to have swung the other way. According to the National Center for Health Statistics, the divorce rate in the U.S. dropped to 4.7 per 1,000 people at the beginning of the decade. Economic considerations, the fear of AIDS, a general maturing of the baby-boom generation—all these factors have been offered to account for the drop. While they have probably contributed, a more fundamental factor seems to be having even more effect: people are realizing that making commitments and keeping promises is at the heart of being authentic human beings.

Several states now require parents contemplating divorce to attend seminars on how divorce will affect their children. The courses usually consist of lectures, films, and role playing to dramatize the conflicts that complicate the lives of people following divorce. After these court-mandated sessions, some couples drop their divorce proceedings and seek help in rebuilding their marriages. In other words, our culture is beginning to look at itself and see the unpleasant realities it has generated. It is looking for an alternative to self-centeredness, the breakdown of the family, and the hopelessness that leads to drugs or other criminal behaviors among its children. These are spiritual problems and cannot be solved without the redemptive message of Christ.

Are there marriages that simply will not work? Certainly so. But far too many people walk away from marriages that could be saved. Unwilling to invest the energy necessary for self-understanding and improvement of a relationship, they throw in the towel. They then proceed to establish a new marriage—between 70 and 75 percent of divorced persons will remarry—that will fail because of the same unaddressed and unresolved issues that undid the previous one.

The seventh commandment is about marriage. Specifically, it is an attempt to keep marriages intact by forbidding adultery. Marriage is not a prerequisite to being within the will of God; for anyone who does marry, however, the will of God requires that he or she honor and keep the holy covenant made before God. To fail to do so is to be guilty of a sin with fearful consequences for all parties involved.

THE *COVENANT* NATURE OF MARRIAGE

Since this commandment is designed to protect marriage, an investigation of its significance must start with a review of what the Bible says about the married state. Both Old and New Testaments are full of positive teaching on honoring one's commitment in marriage.

By definition, marriage is a covenant between a man and woman that is to be lived in love until death separates them. The verse that supplies the substance of this definition is found in the opening lines of the Bible, at the end of the creation account. After relating how Yahweh created a woman and brought her to the first man, the account is closed with this generalization about all husband-wife unions: "For this reason a man will leave his father and mother and be united to his wife, and they will become one flesh" (Gen. 2:24).

As John R. W. Stott has pointed out, this verse implies that a marital commitment is *exclusive* ("a man . . . his wife . . ."), *publicly signified* in some culturally approved manner ("will leave his father and mother"), *lasting* ("be united to his wife"), and *consummated by sexual intimacy* ("become one flesh"). In the light of factors at work in our culture today, a fifth implication may need to be expounded. That marriage is between "a man" and "his wife" signifies its nature as a *heterosexual* relationship.

This verse does not say that marriage is irrevocable, for we shall shortly find that divorce is allowed under certain limited circumstances. Yet it is obvious in Scripture that dissolving a marriage is always a departure from God's ideal will. Marriage is meant to be a lifelong relationship.

Jesus verifies this analysis of the Genesis text. In responding to a question about divorce from some Pharisees who approached him, he began with an affirmation about the nature of marriage.

"Haven't you read," he replied, "that at the beginning the Creator 'made them male and female,' and said, 'For this reason a man will leave his father and mother and be united to his wife, and the two will become one flesh'? So they are no longer two, but one. Therefore what God has joined together, let man not separate." (Matt. 19:4–6)

From the words of Jesus, then, it is obvious that the divine intention of permanence is inherent in the marriage covenant. As the traditional language of a marriage ceremony puts it, this relationship "is not to be entered into thoughtlessly but soberly and in the fear of God."

The prophetic books of the Old Testament offer several statements that are critical to our discussion. In reprimanding Judah for the twofold sin of religious and social faithlessness, the prophet Malachi said:

Have we not all one Father? Did not one God create us? Why do we profane the covenant of our fathers by breaking faith with one another?

Judah has broken faith. A detestable thing has been committed in Israel and in Jerusalem: Judah has desecrated the sanctuary the LORD loves, by marrying the daughter of a foreign god. As for the man who does this, whoever he may be, may the LORD cut him off from the tents of Jacob—even though he brings offerings to the LORD Almighty.

Another thing you do: You flood the LORD's altar with tears. You weep and wail because he no longer pays attention to your offerings or accepts them with pleasure from your hands. You ask, "Why?" It is because the LORD is acting as the witness between you and the wife of your youth, because you have broken faith with her, though she is your partner, the wife of your marriage covenant.

Has not the LORD made them one? In flesh and spirit they are his. And why one? Because he was seeking

> godly offspring. So guard yourself in your spirit, and do not break faith with the wife of your youth.
>
> "I hate divorce," says the LORD God of Israel, "and I hate a man's covering himself with violence as well as with his garment," says the LORD Almighty.
>
> So guard yourself in your spirit, and do not break faith. (Mal. 2:10–16)

Note the straightforward statement of God's hatred of divorce. For now, the issue of significance in this section of Holy Scripture is the covenant principle signified by marriage. Verse 14 speaks of the "marriage *covenant*," and a Hebrew verb translated "breaking faith" is used five times (2:10, 11, 14, 15, 16) to describe the faithlessness of people in relation to their covenants.

Yahweh's unique relationship with Jerusalem is described at some length in another prophetic book under the figure of marriage. In that extended text, the word "covenant" is again the pivotal term. "I gave you my solemn oath and entered into a covenant with you, declares the Sovereign LORD, and you became mine" (Ezek. 16:8b). But the people were guilty of "prostitution" by going after idols. Thus they were to be sentenced to the "punishment of women who commit adultery" (Ezek. 16:38a). All this would happen "because you have despised my oath by breaking the covenant" (Ezek. 16:59b).

Even in a poetic section of the Old Testament, a woman's marriage is "the covenant she made before God" with a man (Prov. 2:17). Thus it is clear that the essence of the relationship called marriage is covenanting: it is promising faithfulness and guaranteeing loyalty; it is committing oneself and pledging allegiance. As with every covenant, mutual rights and responsibilities come with marriage. Since this covenant relationship was created by God and because individual marriage covenants are made before him, married persons have a relationship that extends beyond two humans to involve God himself.

These biblical references combine to explain how marriage is meant to work and to identify the ideal for male-female commitments within wedlock. God is love, and all his actions toward his people are self-giving. Yahweh made a covenant with the ancient Hebrews; and even when they broke their commitments and failed to live up to their responsibilities, he continued loving, blessing, and keeping his promises. Christ has made a covenant with his church; and even when we break our commitments and fail to live up to our responsibilities, he continues loving, blessing, and keeping his promises.

The essence of the relationship called marriage is covenanting: it is promising faithfulness and guaranteeing loyalty; it is committing oneself and pledging allegiance.

Is this not the ideal pattern for our marriages, even in their low moments? A woman may realize she has married a clod. A man may discover that his wife is less than the angel he thought she was. With whatever reason each sees for quitting, the divine example counsels loving, blessing, and keeping promises. Hopeful and persevering love honors the covenant and works for healing and growth.

Having offered the divine example of tenacity, the fact remains that some marriages fail beyond hope of repair. Did not God ultimately turn away from national Israel because of her infidelities? Does the New Testament not warn both individuals (cf. 1 Cor. 10:12) and local churches (cf. Rev. 2:5) that they can lose their covenant privileges? If "divorce" is a possibility between God and people he has accepted into covenant relationship, we should not be surprised to find that marital covenants are sometimes dissolved by divorce.

THE DIVORCE LEGISLATION OF SCRIPTURE

When marriage originated in Eden, divorce was not a likely event and remarriage was not an option. This original situation typifies what all marriages should be. From their wedding day forward, bride and groom ought to have eyes for each other only. But the ideal environment of Eden did not survive for long. Neither did the ideal of marriage as a lifelong covenant of self-giving love succeed in escaping the impact of sin.

The corruption of marriage was one of the specific sins that brought about the intolerable depravity of Noah's generation (Gen. 6:1–3). After the flood, another rapid deterioration from the divine ideal for marriage was the background for Abram's fear for his life. He was justifiably afraid that a despot would murder him in order to take the beautiful Sarai into his harem (Gen. 12:10 ff.). Concubinage (Gen. 16:1 ff.), homosexuality (Gen. 19:1 ff.), incest (Gen. 19:30–38), and other sins against marriage produced a gloomy moral climate. What Jesus would later ascribe to the fact that men's "hearts were hard" caused marital fidelity to fall into disrepute and divorce to flourish (cf. Matt. 19:8).

Under the Law of Moses, Yahweh regulated divorce by instituting the "certificate of divorce" (Heb., *get*). Its specific purpose was not to create the institution of divorce but to regulate something already in place in the society; it prohibited a man from remarrying a woman whom he had previously divorced who had since married another man.

> If a man marries a woman who becomes displeasing to him because he finds something indecent about her, and he writes her a certificate of divorce, gives it to her and sends her from his house, if after she leaves his house she becomes the wife of another man, and her second husband dislikes her and writes her a certificate of divorce, gives it to her and sends her from his house, or if he dies, then her first husband, who divorced her, is not allowed to marry her again after she has been defiled. That would be detestable in the eyes of the LORD. Do not bring sin upon the land the LORD your God is giving you as an inheritance (Deut. 24:1–4).

This regulation was surely designed to curb hasty divorce by requiring a legitimate cause for initiating a divorce action, requiring that the matter be brought before a public official, and requiring that a legal document be prepared. The time and effort involved in these formalities served to encourage people to pursue divorce deliberately rather than in the passion of anger.

A hotly contested issue among interpreters of Moses was the meaning of "*something indecent* about her." The Hebrew words behind this translation literally mean "nakedness of a thing" and seem to refer to some sort of sexual misconduct. Debate over the precise meaning raged for centuries. It finally resolved itself to the competing interpretations of Rabbis Hillel and Shammai. The former insisted that the words should be understood in a broad sense that would embrace conduct ranging from sexual infidelity to burning the bread; this view gave rise to the position that a man could "divorce his wife for any and every reason" (Matt. 19:3). The latter argued that the words should be taken in their customary and narrower sense of sexual misconduct; this school of interpretation insisted that divorce should be permitted only in the case of sexual infidelity.

Jesus injected himself into this controversy and sided with the interpretation of Shammai (Matt. 5:31–32). Furthermore, when he was not merely interpreting Moses but giving the divorce legislation that would govern his own disciples, he used precisely the same language to call divorce that had not been occasioned by marital unfaithfulness "adultery" (Matt. 19:9).

Thus both Old and New Testaments are firm in their insistence that marriage is a covenant to be honored. In the case of any divorce, sin is involved. If one has been faithful to his or her covenant only to be betrayed by a partner's sexual transgression, only the betrayer is an adulterer by virtue of getting a divorce. If a couple simply gives up and gets a divorce for a lesser cause, neither walks away completely free of stain.

Since marriage is a covenant-making project, adultery is its covenant-breaking antithesis. The breaking of any promise is wrong. But the dissolution of this most fundamental of all promises between two human beings is especially horrible in the eyes of God. Do you recall the statement cited earlier that summarizes the divine feeling toward divorce? "I hate divorce" are the words of Yahweh cited in Malachi 2:16. He still does. And so does anyone who has witnessed or lived through the anguish of one.

But what about forgiveness for adultery? The person who has honored his or her marriage covenant only to be betrayed by a partner has pain but not guilt to confront. All other persons who divorce have not only pain but guilt to deal with. Their act of breaking a marital covenant makes them adulterers. That this sin, terrible as it may be, is nonetheless forgivable is clear from the teaching of Paul. Notice in particular the italicized portions of the following quotation:

> Do not be deceived: Neither the sexually immoral nor idolaters nor *adulterers* nor male prostitutes nor homosexual offenders nor thieves nor the greedy nor drunkards nor slanderers nor swindlers will inherit the kingdom of God. *And that is what some of you were. But you were washed,* you were sanctified, you were justified in the name of the Lord Jesus Christ and by the Spirit of our God. (1 Cor. 6:9–11)

Our role is not merely to curse the darkness and to announce condemnation of those who have acted outside the divine will. Instead, we teach the judgment of God against all sin—including divorce—and call for repentance. We also help people come to the self-awareness and spiritual insight necessary to move ahead with their lives after divorce. Following the lead of Paul, we tell married people not to divorce (1 Cor. 7:10, 12–14) and counsel the divorced to work toward reconciliation where possible (1 Cor. 7:11). But we also accept that we do not have the final word about others' lives, that they must make their own decisions about human relationships, and that remarriage by divorced persons does not relegate them to second-class citizenship in the kingdom of God (1 Cor. 7:28). God wants people who have failed in a marriage commitment, who have repented and received forgiveness for that failure, and who want to move on with their lives within his will to find encouragement and support from his people rather than condemnation.

FIGHTING FOR OUR MARRIAGES

People who are married need to be on guard constantly against things that threaten fidelity. Couples need to develop "marriage insurance" by a strategy that keeps them alert to the common hazards that sink relationships. Then, if trouble does arise, they need to be humble enough to admit the need for help and to seek spiritual counsel from a trusted source.

Some married people wind up paying a high price because they arrogantly thought they did not have to protect their hearts and behaviors from temptation. For example, today's business world seems to think nothing about travel and after-hours social events where married people are in intimate situations with people other than their mates. At the very least, this constitutes a potential hazard to marital fidelity. Allowing oneself to be in such a position is often a failure to take seriously the Bible's teaching about avoiding situations that tempt us to do evil.

It is no revelation to anyone that our culture has fallen victim to a deliberate flaunting of immorality and contempt for sexual fidelity within marriage. Novels, television, and movies glorify flirtation and justify unfaithfulness. People who value their marriage will have to deliberately resist these messages.

More than these defensive strategies, however, couples who intend to build stable and happy relationships must take a positive approach to strengthening their marriages. Ed Wheat, in his book *Love Life for Every Married Couple,* offers a four-part prescription for what he calls the "best" of all possible marriages. While no human formula for marriage is anything other than an encouragement toward the divine ideal, Wheat offers insights that could help most marriages.

In his scheme, each letter of the word "best" stands for a type of behavior appropriate to people who want to build a strong marriage: blessing, edifying, sharing, and touching.

Blessing your mate means speaking well of her or him. It involves things so simple as saying "Thank you" for little courtesies. Blessing your husband or wife includes kind deeds, saying how much you appreciate the good qualities you see in your partner, and praying to God for him or her.

Edifying simply means building up or encouraging one's mate. This happens when you support your mate in achieving a goal that is important to her, praising how well he does certain things around the house, or responding positively to your mate's attempts at showing love and affection.

Sharing signifies doing things together. Perhaps you enjoy the same sort of exercise or entertainment. Maybe you like to take long walks. But it is even more important that you share conversation, feelings, romantic times, decisions, and spiritual experiences.

Touching denotes all forms of nonsexual contact between a husband and wife—holding hands while walking, a kiss as you part in the morning, gentle pats and hugs when you pass each other in the hall. These are nonverbal statements of your mate's importance and desirability to you.

There are many positive helps for people today who are feeling some degree of disaffection or restlessness in their marriage. There are books to read, tapes to hear, and seminars to attend. There are churches with strong family ministries. There are Christian counselors and marriage therapists. Explore any or all of these as alternatives to breaking your marital covenant. The heartache of countless witnesses stands as a warning to you. God's way of faithful monogamy is still right—both ethically and practically—for people of all times and places. Adultery is often such a devastating experience that it is impossible to recoup the relationship or bear the resulting guilt. A healthy fear of temptation coupled with a strategy for constant improvement of your marriage will pay dividends into eternity.

CONCLUSION

Against the skeptical mood of our time toward marriage, the following facts emerged from a Gallup poll on "Love and Marriage" for the magazine *Psychology Today.* Over 60 percent of American couples say their marriage is "very happy." Fully 90 percent of married people have had only one sexual partner since they got married. Over 80 percent of all married men, regardless of age, say their wife is good-looking. Seventy-five percent of married couples in America say their spouse is their best friend. Eight of ten married persons say they would marry the same person if they had the decision to make over again.

Wondering about making a marriage commitment? Wondering if your marriage can survive a challenge it is facing? Contrary to popular sentiment, the odds are on your side.

By the way, the same Gallup research identified the best predictor of whether or not a couple has a happy marriage: they pray together. The presence of the God who gave Moses commandments on Mount Sinai in the home you are building is the surest way to find stability, joy, and fidelity.

QUESTIONS FOR ADDITIONAL REFLECTION

1. How has divorce affected your family? Personal friends of yours? Your church?
2. Why do you think the Old Testament prophets used adultery as a metaphor for idolatry? How are the two alike?
3. Why would Rabbi Hillel argue for such a broad interpretation of "something indecent" in understanding Deuteronomy 24?
4. Is divorce in a special category of sin, or can it be forgiven as other sins are? Do people ever treat divorce as a different kind of sin? If so, how?
5. How should our churches support and encourage people who have sinned by divorcing their mates and have later repented?
6. What are some situations you face that are dangerous to your marriage?
7. How do you and your mate work to strengthen your marriage?
8. What new approaches could you take toward making your marriage better?
9. Given the "best" formula for marriages referred to in the chapter, is your mate best at blessing, edifying, sharing, or touching? Which do you do best for your spouse?
10. How often do you pray with your mate? What difference does it make in your relationship?

You shall not steal.

Exodus 20:15

CHAPTER TEN

TAKING WHAT BELONGS TO ANOTHER

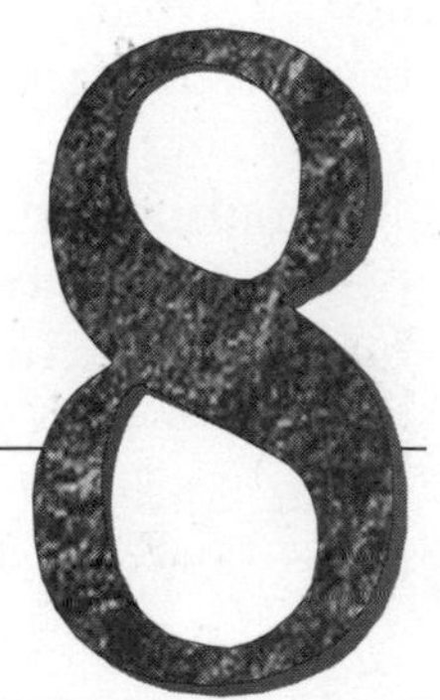

"You shall not steal."

An armored car had collected cash from twenty banks in the San Francisco Bay area and was on its way to the home office of its company. The back door somehow came open and bags of money began to fall out. It was several blocks later when a horn-honking motorist alerted the driver that something was wrong. Before the driver could retrace his route, a traffic jam had been created by people stopping, picking up bags of money, and racing off.

Luis Lopez emerged from the episode a hero. A television repairman, he picked up two bags containing $20,050 each and took them directly to a nearby office of the armored car company whose logo was on the bags. Many more people were thieves rather than heroes, for something over $500,000 was unaccounted for. A police officer said of Mr. Lopez: "While everyone else was busy grabbing what they could get, he was thinking of getting the money back to its rightful owner."

Robbery is the most prevalent crime that Americans have to fear from strangers. It is estimated that muggings, heists at automated teller machines, and other forms of theft occur 1.2 million times each year. In approximately one-third of these instances, the victim is left injured. Property crimes have risen from 1,726 reported crimes per 100,000 persons in 1960 to 4,903 in 1992.

Stealing another's property is a violation of one's fundamental obligation to love others and treat them as he would want to be treated. It is an encroachment on someone else's rights and property. It is taking something under another's authority and possession away from her, depriving her of a rightful possession.

A BIBLICAL ETHIC OF PROPERTY

Collectivism in Scripture?

Contrary to the claims of some, Christianity does not envision the abolition of private property and a collective ownership of possessions. It is true that Acts 4:32–37 tells how the earliest Christians "shared everything they had" and met the needs of certain brothers and sisters by selling possessions and using the proceeds to care for them. But this was not a uniform redistribution of wealth. It was, instead, a voluntary sharing of goods with poor and needy saints. The Jerusalem church had a "daily distribution of food" for the sake of certain members, widows in particular (Acts 6:1). From a close reading of the text, it becomes apparent that these provisions were created by a voluntary pooling of goods.

A husband and wife in that church appear to have been impressed by the kudos awarded to the people giving most generously to its fund for the poor, so they hatched a scheme to get attention for themselves. They sold a parcel of land, brought part of its purchase price to the apostles, and said they were giving the full amount. When they presented their gift, they were both struck dead. The indictment against them is critical to our study. They were punished for lying to God, not for keeping property for themselves. Here are the words of Peter from that incident: "Didn't [your land] belong to you before it was sold? And after it was sold, wasn't the money at your disposal? What made you think of doing such a thing? You have not lied to men but to God" (Acts 5:4). Peter acknowledged that these people were under no obligation to divest themselves of private property. After they chose to sell a tract of land, they were under no obligation to give the proceeds of the sale to the church.

> Christianity does not envision the abolition of private property and a collective ownership of possessions.

The Work Ethic

Rather than common ownership of property, the biblical ideal is work, acquisition, and responsible stewardship of material things. "He who has been stealing must steal no longer, but must work, doing something useful with his own hands, that he may have something to share with those in need" (Eph. 4:28).

God needs men and women of upright character who realize that their earning power is from God and who feel a strong sense of responsibility to use their wealth for holy purposes in this world. Wealth is not equivalent to virtue, nor is poverty a vice. Some evil people accumulate fortunes, and some godly persons go bankrupt. If God has prospered you and allowed you to become wealthy, acknowledge everything you have as his gift to you and be unselfish in its use. Realize that God's work in the world can be enlarged by your generosity. On the other hand, if you have not been as fortunate and prosperous as someone else, don't resent that person or compromise your integrity in trying to "get a slice of the pie." It is what you have in your heart rather than your hand that establishes your status before God.

Because some hearts are corrupt, greedy, and selfish, there will always be people who try to acquire property dishonestly. Public officials have been known to use their positions for personal profit—soliciting bribes, taking kickbacks, etc. Retail stores are estimated to lose approximately ten billion dollars per year in retail pilferage and shoplifting. People hide income from the Internal Revenue Service and cheat on their tax returns. Whatever the form, stealing is always wrong.

Stewardship

The Bible teaches believers to view their relationship to property and wealth as a *stewardship.* In Jesus' Parable of the Talents (Matt. 25:14–30), he told the story of a man who went away on a trip. In his absence, the management of his property was entrusted to various servants. Upon his return, there was a time of accountability when each was required to explain how he had used his master's possessions. Servants who had been given five and two talents respectively doubled their master's investment; the servant entrusted with one talent brought only the original amount and returned no profit. The two productive servants were rewarded, and the unproductive one was called a "wicked, lazy servant."

The point of this parable is hardly ambiguous. Our Master has gone away for a time. In his absence, various things have been entrusted to his servants. We have different degrees of ability, wealth, education, influence, etc. While the Master is away, we are expected to use whatever he has left to us to honor him and promote his interests among humankind. When he returns, there will be a time of accountability. We will answer to him as people who have held his possessions in trust.

Under American civil law, one may either own property or hold another's goods in trust. Under divine law, everything under a human being's authority is regarded as God's property held in trust.

Whatever is entrusted to a human being is under his or her control for only a short time. Jesus expects it to be used with eternity in view.

> "Do not store up for yourselves treasures on earth, where moth and rust destroy, and where thieves break in and steal," he said. "But store up for yourselves treasures in heaven, where moth and rust do not destroy, and where thieves do not break in and steal. For where your treasure is, there your heart will be also." (Matt. 6:19–21)

Paul took up the subject of how wealth should be viewed and wrote:

> Command those who are rich in this present world not to be arrogant nor to put their hope in wealth, which is so uncertain, but to put their hope in God, who richly

> provides us with everything for our enjoyment. Command them to do good, to be rich in good deeds, and to be generous and willing to share. In this way they will lay up treasure for themselves as a firm foundation for the coming age, so that they may take hold of the life that is truly life. (1 Tim. 6:17–19)

From this Pauline text, at least five things should be noted. *First,* people who are wealthy need not feel guilty. Wealth is a gift from God, just like sunshine and good health, and is intended by God to provide "enjoyment" to those who have it. *Second,* wealth incurs guilt for its possessors only when it leads to "arrogance" or selfishness (a refusal to be "generous and willing to share"). *Third,* whatever degree of wealth one has, he or she should remember how "uncertain" it is. *Fourth,* the only secure grounding of one's hope for the future is in God, not in the gathering and investing of money. *Fifth,* people whose spiritual priorities lead them to use their wealth in order to be "rich in good deeds" are following the Lord's command to "lay up treasure" in heaven and have discovered the true meaning of life.

> Under divine law, everything under a human being's authority is regarded as God's property held in trust.

There are things that God wants his people to do in this world that require money. But we are sometimes irresponsible and unspiritual in our stewardship of the funds that we dedicate specifically to his service. It is *not* a requirement of faith, for example, that churches build expensive worship facilities. It *is* an obligation of the Christian religion, however, that we evangelize the world (Matt. 28:19–20) and care for the poor (Matt. 25:34–36). Are Christians faithful to God when they erect great church building monuments and have no missions program? Is a church that spends less than 5 percent of its budget on helping the poor exhibiting right priorities?

The temptation for any individual or group is to view prosperity either as an end in itself or as a means to self-gratification. This view is a far cry from the biblical ethic of stewardship. Thus the warning of Scripture:

> But godliness with contentment is great gain. For we brought nothing into the world, and we can take nothing out of it. But if we have food and clothing, we will be content with that. People who want to get rich fall into temptation and a trap and into many foolish and harmful desires that plunge men into ruin and destruction. (1 Tim. 6:6–9)

Always wanting more than one has (or more than someone else has) can create the desire to deprive others of what they have. This insatiable appetite for more leads to dishonesty, deception, and stealing. Murder, prostitution, gambling, drug trafficking, broken contracts, lying, and every imaginable evil can be traced to someone's selfish greed. "For the love of money is a root of all kinds of evil," said Paul. "Some people, eager for money, have wandered from the faith and pierced themselves with many griefs" (1 Tim. 6:10).

The antidote to greed in the life of a believer is generosity. The Old Testament required Israelites to offer a variety of tithes and gifts to God as worship. According to the estimates of some scholars, these requirements would have equaled between one-fourth and one-third of a person's annual income. Christians are not assigned an amount or percentage to give the Lord but are told simply to be liberal in their offerings (Rom. 12:8b). One who cultivates a generous spirit will not fall prey to the lust for money.

The antidote to greed in the life of a believer is generosity.

VIOLATING THIS COMMANDMENT

At least four categories of action come to mind that constitute clear violations of the eighth commandment. All are forms of stealing that take for oneself what properly belongs to another.

Taking Money or Property from Another

Taking money or tangible property that is not rightfully one's own is stealing. This is the most obvious form of theft and has been talked about already in this chapter. Burglary, embezzlement, fraud, plagiarism—all are forms of theft, but so are padded expense accounts and bogus insurance claims. Contracting debts beyond one's reasonable ability to pay or simply leaving a debt unpaid is a form of stealing.

A New York City high school student found a purse and turned it in—complete with one thousand dollars in cash. Not a single school official congratulated her on her upright behavior. "If I come from a position of what is right and wrong," said her teacher, "then I am not [her] counselor." What can such an ethically garbled statement mean? Apparently it translates to something like this: "All things are relative, and we no longer believe that anything is right or wrong." We can only hope that the number of people teaching and modeling such cynical value judgments before our young people are few and far between.

Dishonesty in Business Dealings

Failing to give full value in one's business dealings is stealing. In ancient days, people had to be wary of merchants who kept two sets of weights in their equipment. They would buy with the use of a set of heavy weights, thus getting a premium for themselves. Then they would sell with their light weights, thereby holding back from their clients. This greatly increased their margins of profit when trading in wheat or some other product. This sort of conduct was explicitly condemned among Yahweh's covenant people, for it was a form of dishonesty and stealing (Deut. 25:13–15). Today's equivalent practices of overpricing goods and services or misrepresenting the quality of a product is no less dishonest.

An employer's refusal to pay fair wages or to honor bonus clauses steals from the people working for him. On the other hand, an employee is guilty of stealing from the person who hired him by failing to put in the hours or perform the tasks that were accepted. Either behavior is wrong (cf. Eph. 6:5–9; James 5:4).

Taking Intangible Things from Another

One may be guilty of stealing by taking intangible things from others. One of the cruelest and most ungodly forms of stealing from another is to deny his or her rights in society. A flood of legislation has been passed since the 1960s to secure and safeguard the civil rights of women, Afro-Americans, Hispanics, and other minorities in the United States. As we approach the dawn of the twenty-first century, sexism, racism, and other forms of discrimination are still commonplace.

Perhaps the most common way one steals an intangible from another is through gossip and slander.

To deny housing, education, jobs, or other opportunities to someone because of skin color, ethnic background, or sex is sinful. Many a female, however, knows that in many situations she will likely be paid considerably less money than a male for doing the exact same work. Statistics about the number of women and blacks in management positions with America's leading corporations make the concept of a "glass ceiling" believable. Legislation will never end all the inequities and discriminations we have created. It will take a stronger force than law to change attitudes and behavior patterns held over from earlier times. It will take the power of Christian love. It is wrong to steal rights and respect from beings who are created in the image of God, and it is right to use your influence to challenge such injustices wherever you see them.

Perhaps the most common way one steals an intangible from another is through gossip and slander. To injure someone by telling lies or spreading misinformation is a wicked violation of this commandment.

Withholding from God

Failing to be generous toward God in one's gifts and offerings is stealing. In the last book of our canonical Old Testament, God asked this question of his people: "Will a man rob God?" He went on to affirm that Israel had done just that. Anticipating that the people would ask how that was possible, he said they robbed him "in tithes and offerings" (Mal. 3:8). If the failure of the people of God to supply their offerings was stealing under the old covenant, surely it is no less serious an offense under the new.

RESTITUTION: A FORGOTTEN PRINCIPLE

One who has been guilty of violating the commandment against stealing must repent in order to be forgiven. Repentance certainly involves remorse over past evil and a halt to any and all behaviors that constitute theft. But there is another biblical principle, often overlooked, that must be considered a part of repentance.

The civil code of the Old Testament made the obligation of *restitution* clear in all instances where there had been an offense against the eighth commandment. Several specific offenses and the restitution they required are detailed in Exodus 22:1–15. And a general rule about restitution is given in Leviticus 6:1–7. The latter text says that one who had committed an act of robbery was required to offer a guilt offering to the Lord. Before he could take his offering to the priest, however, he had to restore the stolen property (or its replacement value) and add 20 percent to its value as restitution.

The requirement to "add a fifth of the value" upon returning stolen property seems to have been a minimum restitution penalty. In some cases, it was considerably higher. For example, because of their importance to one's economic situation in Israel, stolen sheep or oxen had to be restored four for one, or five for one respectively (Exod. 22:1).

During the personal ministry of Jesus, he encountered a man at Jericho named Zacchaeus. As a tax collector, he shared the fate of fellow tax collectors: he was an outcast from polite society. But Jesus went to his house and spoke with him about the kingdom of God. At the end of their visit, Zacchaeus was moved to say, "Look, Lord! Here and now I give half of my possessions to the poor, and if I have cheated anybody out of anything, I will pay back four times the amount" (Luke 19:8). He knew the Law of Moses well enough that he understood dishonesty could be forgiven only when restitution was made for the offense.

Our civil laws could be made far more just by incorporating this principle. Much of the overcrowding in our prisons could be relieved by putting men and women who have committed property crimes to work outside the prison walls, with a court-ordered obligation to restore and compensate those who were victimized by their actions. Why should taxpayers house thieves and thus be victimized by them again? Wouldn't it be fairer for the ones who have done harm against property to support themselves, replace what they stole, and pay compensation to those who suffered by their actions? Our present prison system puts violent persons, whose original crimes were against people (mugging, rape, murder), back onto the streets much too soon. Keep the violent offenders in jail, and let those whose offenses were against property work on the outside, be accountable under parolee-type supervision, and put a portion of their earnings into a restitution fund. Our present method of criminal justice often brutalizes people who are incarcerated and offers nothing to the people who were originally harmed by them.

Our civil laws could be made far more just by incorporating the principle of restitution.

Personal relationships should also honor the principle of restitution. Saying "I'm sorry" is a proper beginning point in cases of gossip, violated trust, and the like; but it does not undo, repair, or compensate the harm that may have been inflicted. Often, in fact, the harm cannot be undone. At the very least, however, people should set the record straight by informing those to whom they have lied of the truth. They should have the courage to return something that belongs to another and compensate any losses that were incurred by its rightful owner.

CONCLUSION

There is an old folktale about honesty that bears retelling in modern times. Adults, as well as children, need to learn its lesson.

Once upon a time, a lazy man decided to sneak into his neighbors' fields and steal grain for himself. "If I take only a little from each field, no one will ever miss it," he told himself, "but it will all add up to a great store of grain that will see me through the winter." So he waited for the darkest night, when the light of the moon was completely absent, and he crept out of his house.

He took his young daughter with him. "Daughter," he whispered, "you must stand guard and call out if anyone spies me."

The man crept into the first field and began to reap. Before long the child called out, "Father, someone sees you!"

Frightened, the man looked all around. But he saw no one, so he gathered his stolen cache and moved on to a second field.

"Father, someone is looking!" the child cried again.

Again the man stopped dead in his tracks to look around. Once again he saw nobody. He gathered still more grain and moved to a third field.

A little while passed, and the daughter called out, "Father, someone sees you!"

This time, more annoyed than frightened, he looked around quickly. He saw no one. So he continued to gather grain that had been produced by another's labor.

Coming to the last field, he was ready to begin reaping where he had not sowed. "Father, someone is looking at you!" said the child again.

The thief stopped, looked around carefully, and again found no one. "Why do you keep saying someone sees me?" he asked angrily. "I've looked everywhere, and I don't see anyone."

"Father," said the little girl, "there is Someone who sees you from above."

QUESTIONS FOR ADDITIONAL REFLECTION

1. How would you react if twenty thousand dollars fell from a vehicle in front of your car? What if you knew no one was looking?
2. What is the difference in owning something and holding it in trust? What significance do you see in this distinction for Christian stewardship?
3. How does an eternal perspective change one's view of the priority of material things?
4. What method do you suggest for making spiritual decisions about money that is dedicated to God?
5. How would your lifestyle change if you were required to give one-fourth or one-third of your annual income to God?
6. Four categories of stealing are described in this chapter. Which of those four seems easiest for you to avoid? Which is hardest to avoid?
7. Have your ever considered such things as irresponsible indebtedness, sexism, and slander as forms of stealing? Are they? Justify your answer.
8. How do you feel about incorporating the principle of restitution into our criminal justice system?
9. In light of the various types of stealing discussed in the chapter, is there anyone to whom you need to make restitution?

You shall not give false testimony against your neighbor.

Exodus 20:16

CHAPTER ELEVEN

THE PINOCCHIO SYNDROME

9

"You shall not give false testimony."

The very word *Pinocchio* communicates the issue of truthfulness/lying to most of us because of Carlo Lorenzini's famous story. The story lies behind such rebukes as "Your nose is growing!" when confronting an untruth. In the famous scene during which Pinocchio's nose grows to such humorous lengths, the wooden puppet is asked a question by the Fairy with the Blue Hair.

> "What did you do with the four gold pieces?"
> "I lost them," replied Pinocchio. But he told a lie, because he had them in his pocket. The moment he said this, his nose, which was already long enough, grew four inches longer.
> "Where did you lose them?" asked the Fairy.
> "In the forest near here."
> At this second lie, the nose grew still longer.

> "If you have lost them in the forest near here," said the Fairy, "we shall soon find them. For everything here is always found."
>
> "Ah, now I recollect," said the marionette. "I did not lose the coins, but I swallowed them when I took the medicine."
>
> At the third lie, Pinocchio's nose grew so long that he couldn't turn around. If he turned one way he struck it against the bedpost or the window. If he turned it another, he hit the wall or the door.
>
> The Fairy looked at him and began to laugh.
>
> "Why are you laughing?" asked the marionette sheepishly.
>
> "I laugh at the foolish lies you have told."
>
> "How did you know they were lies?"
>
> "Lies, my boy, are recognized at once, because they are of only two kinds. Some have short legs, and others have long noses. Yours are the kind that have long noses."
>
> Pinocchio was so crestfallen that he tried to run away and hide himself, but he couldn't. His nose had grown so long that he couldn't get through the door.

Unfortunately for those who are deceived and abused by them, people who tell lies can do so without suffering noticeable changes in their physical appearance. Oh, small children or otherwise truthful people may squirm, blush, or somehow give themselves away when they dabble in falsehood, but the people who have learned to lie as a way of life give no obvious sign of their prevarications. With straight faces and earnest tones, crooked politicians, shady sales people, and self-serving religionists say whatever they believe is necessary to get elected, make a sale, or win a convert.

What has become of the premium our culture once placed on truthfulness? Have we abandoned "Is it true?" for "Will it bring about the desired effect?" as the primary self-test for personal affirmations? Has the ninth commandment been repealed?

A NATION OF LIARS?

A national newsmagazine raised the question "Are We a Nation of Liars?" One indicator that supports the claim that we are is America's tabloid press. For example, one carried a rather typical headline: "World's Oldest Newspaper Carrier, 101, Quits Because She's Pregnant." Beside the headline was the photograph of Nellie Mitchell of Mountain Home, Alabama, who promptly sued the Florida-based *Sun* tabloid. As a matter of fact, Ms. Mitchell had once delivered papers. She quit doing so at the age of ninety, and her last pregnancy had been when she was thirty-five. In court testimony, a *Sun* editor revealed that, since the Mitchell photo was taken in 1980, he assumed she was dead and therefore could not be libeled. The paper's attorney said, "Most reasonable people recognize that the stories are essentially fiction." Unmoved by the tabloid's sudden candor about playing fast and loose with the truth, a jury awarded Mitchell $1.5 million in damages.

Government officials have been caught lying often enough that their credibility gets very low marks in national polls on honesty. Scientists have been dismissed from jobs for falsifying research. Workers alter career credentials on job applications to get positions they want. Christians who become embroiled in church fights manufacture and spread falsehoods about their "enemies." One can quickly become cynical by seeing how easily and how often people lie.

Perhaps the younger generation will reverse the trend. But Michael Josephson, head of the Josephson

Institute of Ethics, doubts it. His nonprofit foundation devoted to character education conducted a survey of nearly seven thousand college and high school students in 1991–1992. One-third of the high schoolers and 16 percent of the university students said they had taken an item from a store without paying for it during the previous year. One out of six admitted they had lied on a resume, job application, or during an employment interview. Even more (33 percent) said they were willing to lie on a resume. Thirty percent said they had lied to a customer at least once during the past year.

"There is a hole in the moral ozone," said Josephson, "and it is probably getting bigger." Upon releasing the research cited above, he expressed his belief that unethical behavior is common among the younger generation because adults have been such poor examples and because society fails to impose serious negative consequences for dishonesty.

Then there are the periodic church-sponsored, letter-writing campaigns against Madalyn Murray O'Hair's petition before the Federal Communications Commission to ban religious broadcasting. The FCC has received millions of pieces of mail in opposition to it. The only problem is that Mrs. O'Hair has never filed such a petition. Yet the rumor (euphemism for "lie") has surfaced again and again over the past twenty years. Similar to it are rumors about Liz Claiborne insulting black women on *The Oprah Winfrey Show* (Ms. Claiborne has not been on Oprah's show), the President of Procter & Gamble going public on *The Phil Donahue Show* about using company profits to support the Church of Satan (no such program ever aired), or a report on CBS's *60 Minutes*—or, in another version, ABC's *20/20*—that Wendy's had served hamburger meat mixed with ground red worms (another falsehood). Rumor-mongering is simply another form of lying that attempts to hurt an institution or person with untruths.

The book *The Day America Told the Truth* says that 91 percent of those surveyed lie routinely about matters they consider trivial, and 36 percent lie about important matters. If these statistics are correct, honorable and truthful people are at the mercy of a majority of their dishonorable and untruthful peers.

"WHAT IS TRUTH?"

When Jesus was on trial before Pontius Pilate, there was an interesting exchange between the two about truth. "I came into the world to testify to the truth," said Jesus. "Everyone on the side of truth listens to me." The Roman procurator replied with a cynical question: "What is truth?" (John 18:37–38).

Pilate was a military man who had more recently become a politician. He had probably gotten his appointment to govern the Jewish territory by manipulating the truth and lying. He likely trusted no one among his associates and was on guard constantly against their lies and misrepresentations to him. Now a man standing before him was talking about *the truth.* His cynicism reflects the attitude that, since no one has perfect knowledge and since human intelligence is not infallible, "truth" is only a nonsense word that has no legitimate place in the vocabulary of humans. That attitude has not disappeared.

Factual Truth Versus Moral Truth

In order to get at Pilate's question in a serious way, there are two major aspects of truth that must be explored: factual truth and moral truth.

Factual truth has to do with the accuracy of statements in relation to the state of affairs they allege to describe. A statement is judged "true" if what is said really does represent the state of affairs to which it refers. The statement "That car belongs to John" is a true statement if the car in question really does belong to John; otherwise it is false. The statement "Jesus is the Son of God" is true if and only if Jesus really is who he claims to be; otherwise it is false.

But there is another way to approach the truth subject, and that is in terms of *moral truth.* This has to do with one's honesty in telling the truth and not withholding what he or she believes to be the facts of the matter. Howard tells a caller on the phone "Theresa isn't here." As a matter of fact, Theresa is present and looking Howard in the eye. But he knows Theresa doesn't want to speak to the person who is calling. Or a family and a physician enter into a conspiracy to tell someone in the hospital bed "You don't have cancer" when the surgery just completed has found a malignancy. The people have made the decision to hide the truth they know from the patient.

While the two elements of factual truth and moral truth cannot be totally separated, it is the latter that is primary in the ninth commandment. "You shall not give false witness against your neighbor" does not require you to be omniscient, but it does require you to be honest. It does not demand that you have the full content of factual truth in your possession, but it does require you to be trustworthy when you speak about some matter wherein the facts are in your possession.

In other words, this ethical mandate is not so much about knowledge as it is about veracity, candor, and integrity. Neither God nor man can command "Don't be lacking in information on any subject" or "Don't be perplexed about some difficult matter." But both God and our neighbors have the right to say "Don't tell lies" and "Don't misrepresent facts so as to deceive me, mislead me, or send me down some blind alley."

Personal Integrity

Believers in God must hold personal integrity in the highest regard. If asked about a matter she knows but thinks ought not be revealed, a believer can reply that she is not at liberty to give out that information and refuse to pursue the subject. What she must *not* do is mask what she knows with layers of falsehoods.

Believers must love truth telling and abhor lying in order to honor our likeness to the God in whose image we have been created. God is truthful in word and deed (Rev. 15:3; 16:7). Because of his holy nature, he cannot lie (Titus 1:2; cf. Num. 23:19). Furthermore, the Spirit of God who indwells Christians is himself the "Spirit of Truth" (John 14:17; 1 John 4:6; 5:6). And Jesus Christ is the very personification of truth (John 14:6).

"Therefore each of you must put off falsehood and speak truthfully to his neighbor, for we are all members of one body" (Eph. 4:25). Because humans live in community, it is critical that we be able to depend on the information passed from person to person within the group. We must be able to trust one another, to have confidence in each other's integrity. Lies destroy credibility, and once trust is undermined by lies, half-truths, and deceptions, right relationships are difficult to restore.

In his listing of seven things Yahweh hates, Solomon named two things that relate to trafficking in untruths.

> There are six things the LORD hates, seven that are detestable to him: haughty eyes, *a lying tongue,* hands

> that shed innocent blood, a heart that devises wicked schemes, feet that are quick to rush into evil, *a false witness who pours out lies* and a man who stirs up dissension among brothers. (Prov. 6:16–19)

And among the final lines of the Bible is a stern warning that no one who loves or lives falsehoods can enter heaven. "Outside [God's dwelling] are the dogs, those who practice magic arts, the sexually immoral, the murderers, the idolaters and *everyone who loves and practices falsehood*" (Rev. 22:15).

HOW WE VIOLATE THIS COMMANDMENT

Perjury

The most direct application of the ninth commandment is its prohibition of the legal offense called *perjury.* For one to "give false testimony" is to testify falsely in any sort of formal hearing.

Under the Law of Moses, a severe penalty was imposed on anyone who perjured himself. Deuteronomy 19:15–19 makes it clear that the court was to impose on any perjurer the sentence his lie would have brought to the accused. "If the witness proves to be a liar, giving false testimony against his brother, then do to him as he intended to do to his brother." If a man gave false testimony in a capital case and was exposed, he would pay with his own life; death is the penalty his lie would have brought on an innocent person. If a witness falsely charged someone with stealing another man's sheep, the witness would have to requite the stolen property at the rate of four sheep for each one missing. That is the penalty that would have been imposed on an innocent person if the lie had gone undetected.

Our formulation of this command in the United States is: "Do you solemnly swear to tell the truth, the whole truth, and nothing but the truth, so help you God?" When one responds "I do" to that oath, he or she is under penalty of perjury if the truth is misrepresented in the testimony given.

While the swearing in ceremony in a court is solemn, it ought not be necessary to ask a Christian to verify his word with an oath. Christians regard the truth as sacred always—whether under oath in court or having casual conversation in the church foyer. This fact leads to a second consideration.

All Lying

This commandment also prohibits all lying. It would be far too narrow an application of this rule to limit it only to testimony given in courts and formal hearings. In the Old Testament code of personal conduct, a descendant of Abraham was forbidden ever to lie to his brother: "Do not steal. Do not lie. Do not deceive one another" (Lev. 19:11; cf. Matt. 5:33–37). Lying is a mockery of human kinship, an affront to the character of God, and an attack on the fundamental trust that allows society to move forward.

Perhaps the time has come in this study to be precise in answering the question *"What is a lie?"* Is every untruth a lie? No, for this would include honest mistakes of inaccurate information passed along unwittingly. What about concealment? We are getting closer to a workable definition now, but the definition needs to be more precise. No person ever tells another everything he or she knows; not even God tells everything. He has revealed many things in Scripture, but many more remain in his private possession (Deut. 29:29; cf. Matt. 24:36).

Concealment is a lie only when the thing hidden from others relates to some moral obligation one has to the hearer. For example, Abraham was guilty of lying to Abimelech about Sarah. Because Sarah was so beautiful and because he feared for his life, Abraham said that she was his sister. What he said was true, after a fashion, for she and Abraham had the same father. But in telling only that much about their relationship, Abraham concealed the much more important fact that she was also his wife. In his concealment, he sinned against Abimelech by positioning him to claim Sarah as his wife. Thus Abraham caused Abimelech to commit a moral offense by virtue of what he concealed (Gen. 20:1–18).

Lying is a mockery of human kinship, an affront to the character of God, and an attack on the fundamental trust that allows society to move forward.

On the other hand, there are cases such as the one involving Samuel and King Saul where concealment is not wrong. Wicked Saul had become defensive of his throne and bitterly jealous of anyone who represented a threat to his rule. When God rejected Saul and told the prophet Samuel to go down to anoint one of the sons of Jesse as Israel's next king, Samuel was afraid the king would discover his travel plans and ask why he was going to Bethlehem. In effect, Yahweh told him, "Samuel, the king has no business knowing where you are going or what you will do there. I have rejected Saul as king over the nation, and whom I select to replace him is my affair alone. So take an animal appropriate for sacrifice with you so that, if anyone wants to know where you are going and what you intend to do, you can say that you are going to Bethlehem to offer a sacrifice to me. The rest of your mission there is between the two of us alone" (cf. 1 Sam. 16:1–5). Not all concealment, then, is lying. There are some things others have no need or right to know. What you choose to volunteer is your business. Concealment becomes a lie only if what is kept from another is something he or she has the right to know for the sake of some moral obligation.

How, then, shall we define a lie? A lie is *an intentional misleading of another person.* An honest mistake is one thing, but an intentional misrepresentation is something else again.

Slander

The ninth commandment of the Decalogue also forbids slander. "Brothers, do not slander one another," wrote the half-brother of Christ. "Anyone who speaks against his brother or judges him speaks against the law [of love for one's brother, cf. 2:8] and judges it" (James 4:11).

Reference was made earlier to tabloids that play fast and loose with the truth. Perhaps their prevailing commodity is gossip about celebrities. How many stories have been run about Princess Diana? Telling disparaging stories about distinguished people appears to be a fascinating preoccupation with non-Christian people. It is a mean-spirited and wicked use of mental energy, printing presses, and reader time. That the same sort of thing happens so regularly in the religious press and in churches is utterly unthinkable—except for people who know what happens in the Body of Christ.

No religious fellowship—whether the larger brotherhood or a local church—can prosper in an unholy atmosphere that insinuates others' faults and attributes bad motives for apparently praiseworthy deeds. John Calvin spoke of this sin as "fondly exalting ourselves by defaming others." Honest disagreement with a brother or sister is moral; personal abuse of that man or woman in an attempt to undermine credibility is immoral.

THE "JUSTIFIABLE" LIE

As surely as one commits herself or himself to a lifestyle that refuses to deceive or mislead others, someone will ask about "exceptional" cases that appear (to some) to justify lying. What about the biblical case of Rahab protecting the Israelite spies at Jericho by hiding them and lying to the police about their whereabouts? What of a doctor who lies to a terminally-ill patient in order to buoy his spirits? What about government leaders who lie in pursuit of some worthy goal that will benefit national policy? Many insist that lies in these special situations are justifiable.

One who has embraced the fixed and absolute standard of ethics found in Scripture cannot begin allowing exceptions to the obligation of honesty. Once started down the path of rationalization, there is no place to stop. The factors that are supposed to justify "white lies" fail to do so.

The story of Rahab and the spies at Jericho is found in Joshua 2:1–7. Careful reading of the story makes it clear that she was neither complimented nor offered as an example to others for her lies. She was saved by grace through faith, in spite of the fact that she not only lied but was also a prostitute. Hers is a straightforward story of a pagan woman who recognized that the God of the Hebrew nation was the true God. In spite of her immoral sexual history, her willingness to lie in order to deceive the people searching for the Israelite spies, and her very limited knowledge of Yahweh or his covenant, she was saved. The point of this story, then, is not to stamp approval on Rahab's behaviors but to exhibit the loving kindness of Yahweh.

The oft cited case of the physician and her terminal patient hardly offers justification for lying either. A patient has the right to self-determination with regard to his or her body, how to deal with any disease affecting it, and whatever implications follow from that information. To take those rights away from the patient is a paternalistic decision that violates his autonomy as a free person. If the decisions yet to be made do not relate to health care (the disease is too far along for meaningful treatment), they may relate to property disposal, setting limits about future treatment (e.g., "living will" decisions about resuscitation, etc.), clarifying some personal relationships, or settling matters between himself and God. The physician who uses a "benevolent" lie to keep her patient calm may more nearly be protecting herself from the responsibility of having to help him deal with death. Sissela Bok has made this important point about patients' rights to know the truth about their condition:

> Their concern for knowing about their conditions goes far beyond mere curiosity or the wish to make isolated personal choices in the short time left to them; their stance toward the entire life they have lived, and their ability to give it meaning and completion, are at stake.

A government whose leaders manipulate people by paternalistic lies is corrupt and will fail for lack of confidence among its citizens. The recent collapse of Communism in Eastern Europe and the former Soviet Union illustrate this point very well. Repetition of lies did not make the lies believable. The dishonesty of leaders simply caused people to distrust their leadership and mobilized public sentiment to overthrow them. That there is so much distrust of our political leadership in the United States should be of great concern to people who know history's most obvious lessons.

CONCLUSION

This chapter began with a quotation from *Pinocchio.* The puppet had been trapped by his lies, and his nose had grown so that he couldn't get it through the door. What was the resolution of his terrible plight?

> The Fairy let the marionette cry and howl for a good half hour on account of his long nose. She did this in order to teach him a lesson upon the folly of telling falsehoods. But when she saw his eyes swollen and his face red with weeping, she was moved by pity for him. She clapped her hands together, and at the signal a large flock of woodpeckers flew into the window and, alighting one by one upon Pinocchio's nose, they pecked so hard that in a few moments it was reduced to its usual size.

In a culture where truth is so lightly regarded, it is easy for someone to minimize deceptions, half-truths, and outright lies. But lying is not a fine art to be practiced selectively. It is an offense against God and man. There should be a quality of honesty and integrity about Christians—whether in business, professional life, filing an accident report, or simply in casual conversation—that sets them apart. People who follow a God who is always truthful must not excuse themselves for dealing in lies.

QUESTIONS FOR ADDITIONAL REFLECTION

1. Is there a distinction in your mind between lying about trivial matters and lying about important things?
2. Can you illustrate how it is possible to say something that is factually true but morally false?
3. Is it possible to lie by being silent? Can you illustrate how this might happen? Have you ever been guilty of it?
4. Are you inclined to view lying as "immoral" or "against God" in the same way as sexual immorality, murder, and idolatry?
5. Do you agree with the definition of lying offered in this chapter? How might it be improved or made more precise?
6. How are slander and lying related to each other? Is it possible to slander a person if everything you say about him or her is true?
7. What situations might appear to "justify" telling a lie? Is lying ever justified? Why or why not?
8. Imagine for a moment that people's noses actually grow when they tell lies. What would the world around you look like? Would your own appearance be altered?
9. How do you guard your heart against the temptation to lie?

You shall not covet your neighbor's house. You shall not covet your neighbor's wife, or his manservant or maidservant, his ox or donkey, or anything that belongs to your neighbor.

Exodus 20: 17

CHAPTER TWELVE

THE ENVY TRAP

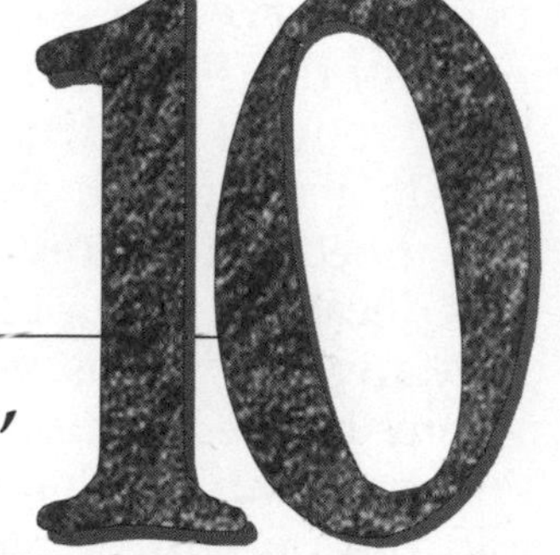

"You shall not covet."

Money is probably envy's most common index. But success in any of its forms is a potential hazardous seduction away from trust in God and toward the counterfeit security of personal self-sufficiency.

When Jesus told his disciples, "How hard it is for *the rich* to enter the kingdom of God!" he might have said the same thing about star athletes, well-educated persons, beautiful women, entertainers, or church leaders. Not all status is measured in dollars; with any form of advantage or privilege comes the danger that the advantage will become more important to the person who has it than the God who gave it.

Lest anyone think, however, that the liability to danger is only to the relatively small percentage of fortunate people who have status, the greater jeopardy is with the large numbers of people who see, lust after, and begrudge the position of others. The '80s will be remembered for such excesses as Malcolm Forbes' garish seventieth birthday bash when eight hundred "close friends" jetted to Morocco for three days of indulgence, Michael Milken's $550 million salary in 1987, Imelda Marcos' three thousand pairs of shoes neatly aligned in her Philippine closet, and Nicolae Ceausescu's practice of importing meat to feed his daughter's dogs while people starved in the Romanian countryside. The hallmark of the '90s, by contrast, may turn out to be diminished returns and frustration as the baby-boom generation is generally unable to attain its high expectations. The greed of the previous decade may thus give way to this decade's envy of those who appear to have more.

Many Christians seem to be trapped in the world's wrong-headed notion of "entitlement." It is no longer enough to affirm that people are entitled to life, liberty, and the pursuit of happiness. The idea is abroad that everyone has the "right" to prosperity and success. But government cannot guarantee prosperity. Schools cannot grant As to everyone. Hospitals cannot provide new hearts, kidneys, and lungs to all whose organs are diseased. The world cannot confer celebrity status on everyone who punts or shoots, sings or acts, writes or paints. And neither Publishers' Clearing House nor the Illinois Lottery can make an instant millionaire of everyone. Thus is created the likelihood that untold numbers of humankind will be trapped in envy.

The final commandment of the Decalogue forbids envy, lust, and unchecked desire. "You shall not covet" strikes at the inner drive that motivates all other evils. People who commit adultery, use religion for leverage against others, steal, or murder first covet.

THE MEANING OF *COVETOUSNESS*

The Bible doesn't teach that it is wrong to dream, work hard, and achieve. Neither does it say that it is wrong to have as much money as someone else or to see something you want, get it, and enjoy its benefits. The sin occurs when the ambition to have or do certain things leads you away from God, corrupts your relationship with your neighbor, destroys your self-control, and diverts you from your responsibilities.

A book titled *The Day America Told the Truth* reported on a national survey that asked adults what they would be willing to do for ten million dollars. One out of four people sampled said they would abandon their families. Almost the same percentage (23 percent) said they would become prostitutes for a week.

A survey of 2,013 members of the active and employed U.S. labor force conducted by the Project on Religion and Economic Values at Princeton University revealed that 68 percent said that money and morality are separate issues. Money and morality can be separated? Success and spirituality are unrelated? The majority may think so, but the Bible says not.

Money is not evil, but the "love of money" is (1 Tim. 6:10). Health, popularity, and influence are not bad things—not one of them is condemned in Scripture. But to define human worth in terms of any or all of them is evil. And to live one's life in pursuit of one or more of them to the neglect of Christ, relationships, family, or integrity is evil.

Sacrificing things of eternal value for a handful of trinkets that cannot be carried into eternity is foolish. To sell your soul for the fool's gold of this world is to make a poor deal. To look down on, mistreat, or withhold compassion from the people who are at the bottom of the world's "ladder of success" is to compromise your own humanity.

Jesus met a man one day who had all the things most people envy. He was young, popular, powerful, and rich. When that man asked the Lord about eternal life, Jesus told him to sell everything he had and give it to the poor. Talk about getting a shock! And when the man decided his bank accounts and land holdings meant more to him than the kingdom of God, his fate was sealed (Luke 18:18–30). So is ours, if anything means more to us than God.

The Hebrew word translated "covet" *(hamad)* in Exodus 20:17 refers to enthusiastic desire. The word itself is morally neutral. That is, one can enthusiastically desire a good thing as well as a bad one. You can have an overwhelming desire to serve God, alleviate hunger, or make your husband happy. There is certainly no vice in these desires. Only when our strong human desires are misdirected toward evil things or get so out of control (even for a good thing) that they turn us away from the divine will are they wrong.

BIBLICAL CASE STUDIES

The attitude of King Ahab toward the vineyard of Naboth is a biblical incident that illustrates the sin of covetousness (1 Kings 21:1–16). Naboth had a prime vineyard that adjoined some of the king's land, and Ahab wanted it for his own. Wanting a piece of valuable property is not sinful. Go to the owner, offer to buy it, and pay him a fair price. That is simply a business transaction and involves no sin.

In this case, however, Naboth did not want to sell his land. It was a family inheritance, and he wanted to pass it on to his heirs. If the story had ended here, no sin would have been committed.

But Ahab's desire for the piece of land quickly got out of control. He went home, lay on his bed, turned his head to the wall, and pouted. His monstrous wife, Jezebel, found out the cause of his unhappiness and took charge. She had Naboth murdered, and Ahab simply went and seized the vineyard he wanted.

A king's greed was so consuming that he was willing to go beyond what was normal, proper, or moral to have his way. But before he and his wife murdered and stole, they coveted.

An incident from the life of an earlier king in Old Testament history shows that one can covet not only money or property but a person (2 Sam. 11:1 ff.). David saw and was smitten by the beauty of Bathsheba. He sent servants to bring her into his palace. Then, even though he found out she was already married to a man named Uriah, he seduced her and committed adultery with her.

David's desires were not held in check. He violated the command against coveting another person's mate. His unrestrained passion resulted in an illicit love affair, murder, and the division of a nation.

A statement in Proverbs 21 makes it clear that one can be covetous without ever becoming a thief, adulterer, or murderer. This verse may, in fact, point to the most common form of covetousness.

> The sluggard's craving will be the death of him, because his hands refuse to work. All day long he craves for more, but the righteous give without sparing (vv. 25–26).

A "sluggard" is one who has lost self-discipline and who therefore fails to fulfill his responsibilities. That such a fate has come upon him is due to his unchecked "craving" (covetousness). By way of a device known as parallelism, verse 26 contrasts his selfish craving for more with a righteous person's generosity. Covetous people evade duty and expect others to carry their weight; in contrast, the industrious person finds joy in giving to others.

Twice in the New Testament, Paul writes that covetousness is a form of idolatry (Eph. 5:5; Col. 3:5). It is the worship of self, for it pledges all of one's energies to self-gratification. It is thus the ultimate of idolatries, for it never allows one to get outside the confining world of self-interest.

Covetousness is the worship of self, for it pledges all of one's energies to self-gratification.

WHAT TO DO WITH GOOD FORTUNE

Maybe you heard about the little boy who was greatly impressed by the visit of a missionary to his church. The man and his family were involved in medical missions, and the nine-year-old boy caught and remembered details of the work they were doing in what we sometimes call the Third World. He was so impressed, in fact, that he talked about it for days afterward.

As he was walking down the street with his mother the following Thursday, he told her, "When I grow up and have a lot of money, I'm going to help a missionary. I think I'll use my money to put a whole team of missionaries somewhere. Maybe I'll even build a hospital."

"Are you sure you'll still feel that way when you grow up and have your own money?" asked his mother.

"Oh, I know I will!" he answered. "If I had money right now, I'd show you. But you know I don't have any money."

Just then the boy spotted a dollar bill blowing along the sidewalk. He turned loose his mother's hand and darted ahead to pick it up. Before his mom could get the word "missionary" out of her mouth, the excited child ducked into a store and plinked down his dollar for a package of baseball trading cards.

Does this story parallel the history of maybe three other people in the world? Or thousands? Or maybe millions? Some of us have such noble intentions for the money we *will* have—someday. Then, as it begins to materialize from work and investments, it goes to filling our pockets with hardly ever a thought for the poor, sick, or lost who once were our alleged stimulus for wanting to make money.

Figures released by the U.S. Department of Commerce in 1990 revealed that people with lower incomes give a larger proportion of their income to churches and charities than higher-income individuals. The figures released to support that claim showed that people with annual household incomes under ten thousand dollars gave 2.8 percent of their earnings to charity, while those who made over one hundred thousand dollars a year gave only 2.1 percent.

Maybe the little boy with no money and noble intent who became the little boy with money that was used only for himself is typical of most of us. Did you ever have a similar dream or intent? Is it still intact? Or do you buy toys? The good that one actually does is a happier criterion for judging a life than the good intentions one had (early on!) along the way.

I remember the big pitch of a college recruiter who came to my high school in the spring of 1963. (I had already made up my mind to go to the school he represented.) He rattled off statistics about expected lifetime earnings. His point was that people who get a college education could expect to make x times more money over a lifetime than their non-college-educated peers would make. And he was recruiting for a Christian college.

Fortunately, I had an English teacher who had taken an interest in me during my high school years. She had talked with me about college too. But I don't ever remember Mrs. Oldham saying anything about money. She spoke instead of doing something worthwhile with my life, finding a way to make the world a little better place to live, and doing something that would help others.

I don't often think of the late Mrs. Oldham, I confess. But she came to mind recently when I read this from Richard J. Foster's *Freedom of Simplicity:*

> Do we see a college education, for example, as a ticket to privilege or as a training for service to the needy? What do we teach our teenagers in this matter? Do we urge them to enter college because it will better equip them to serve? Or do we try to bribe them with promises of future status and salary increases? No wonder they graduate more deeply concerned about their standard of living than about suffering humanity.

Maybe it isn't too late for all of us to think again about why we have certain things. Why do you have certain natural gifts and talents? Why do you have the job you have? Why do you have your education? Why do you have money? Why do you have an apartment or house? Why do you have a car? Why do you have access to a particular resource?

If the answers to these questions all come back only in the first person, maybe it would be appropriate to rethink the early programming someone gave you and your present life priorities. In addition to what these things mean for your personal benefit, they are supposed to fit into a divine plan for loving God and loving your neighbor.

The right answers will never come until we are at least willing to challenge ourselves by asking the questions.

PAUL'S PERSONAL CONFESSION

Let's try a little experiment. There is a purpose to it, so just humor me and go along. Okay? Here's the test: *For the next ten minutes, no matter what happens, promise not to scratch your nose.*

While you are keeping your promise, let's do some Bible study about covetousness from the book of Romans. There is an intensely personal section in the epistle where Paul speaks in the first person singular and confesses the spiritual issue that caused him the greatest exasperation. "I would not have known what coveting really was if the law had not said, 'Do not covet,'" the great apostle wrote. "But sin, seizing the opportunity afforded by the commandment, produced in me every kind of covetous desire" (7:7b–8).

By the way, is anybody's nose itching as much as mine right now? It feels like a cluster of crazy nerve endings is shorting out on me. Feels like a fuzzy caterpillar is sitting on the tip of my nose, like a feather is being raked across my nostrils. Oh, well, back to Paul. Just don't scratch.

Paul's words neither say nor imply that covetousness didn't exist before the Law of Moses named and prohibited it. Neither did he claim that there was no good reason for the prohibition. His point is that the Law's "You shall not covet" had been like an alarm clock in his personal experience to awaken desire and lust and envy.

Banning covetousness not only did not eliminate the problem from his life but it made an already existing problem worse! Sin used the opportunity of law's interdiction to make certain desires more powerful in Paul than they had ever been before.

Incidentally, I met a friend for breakfast at a restaurant recently. When I peppered my scrambled eggs, a fog of that pungent stuff went up my nose. Ever have it happen to you? Remember what it felt like? Well, I sat for the next five minutes sneezing, sniffing, and snorting. Couldn't enjoy breakfast for the pepper. It was terribly annoying! Ah, yes, Romans 7. But remember not to scratch your nose as we proceed.

Paul's point is that a commandment—especially when written as a prohibition—can sometimes have the curious effect of stimulating the desire for the very thing it disallows. "No Trespassing" signs almost compel some people to drive down narrow roads. "Wet Paint" signs seem to require an ever-so-slight test with a fingertip. And every parent knows that saying "Turn that music down!" makes a kid practically deaf and in need of raising the volume ever so slightly.

Is anybody else's nose itching as much as mine? I really need to scratch my prickly proboscis, my refractory olfactory, my self-willed smeller! The tickle seems to be spreading across my entire face. But I'm not going to scratch. You can resist the urge, too, can't you?

Paul never says that divine law is meddlesome, wrong, or evil. He simply observes that sin is so tricky that it uses even so good and holy a thing as law to make us feel like we simply must step across some boundary. I don't think he was describing a phenomenon peculiar to him. Aren't we all that way? Don't we all have passions and desires? Don't we all covet (enthusiastically desire) something?

The problem is that these strong desires can be so easily directed toward the wrong people, the wrong things, the wrong situations. We flirt with the devil's devices, and a command of God to avoid certain things becomes almost a dare.

We flirt with the devil's devices, and a command of God to avoid certain things becomes almost a dare.

For it to be otherwise, something must happen in our hearts. That is the most difficult and astonishing thing about the tenth commandment. Obeying commands against murder, adultery, and stealing is so much easier than obeying this one against coveting. Controlling behavior is one thing, and jails can keep people from inflicting such behaviors as murder and stealing on the larger community, but controlling one's emotions, feelings, and desires is something else again. Paul could elsewhere (Phil. 2:6) claim to have been "faultless" in his observance of legalistic righteousness under the Law of Moses—keeping the commandments against murder, adultery, and stealing, as well as the "traditions of the fathers"—yet admit here that his heart was sometimes out of control with the fires of craving, lust, and covetousness.

When the law forbids what the longing fancies, something must happen on the inside of the person.

God must operate on the heart. Those who say the Decalogue is concerned only with regulating the *externals* of human behavior whereas the New Testament goes more deeply to our *attitudes* and *motivations* sell Scripture short. God has always been concerned with the heart as well as the hands, the real personality as well as the responses to stimuli, the inner fountain as well as the things that pour forth.

That is why God not only saves his people but gives them a new internal dynamic for living. In order to give us victory over our desires, he puts his Holy Spirit in his people to transform and renew their minds (cf. Rom. 12:1–2).

Before we explore this divine solution to human lust, though, we'd better all scratch our noses. Some of you are about to panic already and have been wondering if you could survive. See! Paul was right. Forbidding a thing tends to make it the most urgent matter in the world.

As Paul learned from his personal experience, it is possible to keep the commands of the Law of Moses that govern observable conduct without having one's heart under control. Surely this was also the situation with the rich young ruler who came to Jesus claiming to have kept the commandments from his youth. One can look good to others without his or her heart being captive to God. All of us need to have our hearts purified and transformed. But this is such a monumental task that it is beyond any human ability to perform. It takes the work of the Holy Spirit of God to purify a heart of its unfit cravings.

After his personal confession in Romans 7, Paul moves to a grand affirmation of triumph in Romans 8. The victory he claims is not attributed to willpower but to the Holy Spirit. "The mind of sinful man is death, but the mind controlled by the Spirit is life and peace" (v. 6).

THE DOCTRINE OF SELF-DENIAL

The only way the Holy Spirit can work his holy transformation in a believer's life is for that person to *empty* himself for the sake of being *filled* by his presence and power. That is why Jesus commanded the rich young ruler to "sell everything" under his control and give it away. This requirement was a particular application of a universal principle about faith: "If anyone would come after me," said Jesus, "he must deny himself and take up his cross and follow me" (Matt. 16:24).

Paul's experience of self-denial is recounted in Philippians 3:7–9. There he acknowledged that everything he had once thought valuable he now considered "rubbish" for the sake of Jesus Christ. He obeyed the call of Christ that the rich young ruler rejected. He emptied himself so he could be filled by God's presence.

CONCLUSION

Whatever is dearest and most precious to any one of us is precisely what must be given up for Jesus' sake. "If anyone comes to me and does not hate his father and mother, his wife and children, his brothers and sisters—yes, even his own life—he cannot be my disciple" (Luke 14:26).

What are you proudest of in your life? Family name? House? Looks? Car? Boat? Job? Diplomas? Grandchild? Title? Whatever there is about you that could make you feel self-satisfied or better than others is your greatest temptation. Whatever it is, you may already have it in your possession, or perhaps it is the driving passion of your life. *It will more nearly cost you your soul than murder, adultery, or stealing, for it offers itself to you as an idol to be worshiped.*

Only those who follow Christ can be saved. But to follow him is much more than getting baptized, going to church, and having people think well of you. It is emptying yourself. It is giving up everything for Jesus.

The rich must renounce personal opulence to help the poor and fund the ministry of the gospel. A bright and well-educated person must disown arrogance for the sake of serving in humility. A cultured and handsome man must repudiate vanity and serve others without patronizing them. Whatever advantage you have must be used for the sake of the kingdom of God, or it will corrupt you. It will lead you away from God. It will damn you.

Only when our hearts are focused on God rather than self can our lives have spiritual depth. Only when we are liberated from greed, envy, and covetousness for this world can we be captivated and drawn to the one to come.

QUESTIONS FOR ADDITIONAL REFLECTION

1. Name the form of success that is most attractive to you from this list: money, athletic ability, intelligence, physical attractiveness, fame, power, or some other. Why does it attract you?

2. What might you be tempted to do for ten million dollars?

3. What things do you think about and desire most? Are they holy things or things that have the potential to lead you away from God?

4. Do your personal desires ever compete with God's will? How? What do you do about the conflict?

5. Have you ever had an experience like that of the little boy who found money on the street? Have you given up any of your early, idealistic dreams of sacrifice for the kingdom of God?

6. Why do you have the things you have? Are they for God's purposes or your own? Do you act consistently with your answer?

7. Did you make it through ten minutes without scratching your nose? How difficult was it for you? Did you get the point of the illustration?

8. How has God's Holy Spirit worked to transform and renew your mind?

9. What do you still need to let go of in order to "deny yourself" and follow Christ?

10. Do you agree with the statement that covetousness "will more nearly cost you your soul than murder, adultery, or stealing"? Why or why not?

Righteousness exalts a nation, but sin is a disgrace to any people.

Proverbs 14:34

CHAPTER THIRTEEN

THE ISSUE IS CHARACTER

Concern for an "Ethic of Minimal Civility"

Newspapers carried the word during the 1992 presidential election that Bill Clinton's staff posted signs everywhere reading "It's the economy, stupid!" to keep the campaign agenda focused. As I think about the world we share with one another—suburbs and inner city, female and male, white collar and blue collar, believers and unbelievers—a "little voice" tells me this: *"It's character, stupid! That's the real issue in this world!"*

Maybe millions of bumper stickers and posters with that message need to be posted throughout our social environment. Personal responsibility, concern for others, and commitment to an ethic of minimal civility must be reestablished in American society. The fundamental shift in ethical understanding and behavior that has taken place in recent years must be challenged.

What was once a slow-moving decline of character in the United States has escalated into an avalanche.

A governor of my home state, a vice president of our nation, and a president of the United States of America have been forced out of office in my lifetime because of moral negligence. Insider trading banished Boesky and Milken from Wall Street, and gambling forced Pete Rose out of baseball. The list of names and offenses gets interminably long and depressing.

FAILED ATTEMPTS TO REVERSE ETHICAL DECLINE

As various professions began to suffer in the public eye because of notable ethical lapses, graduate and professional schools began putting courses in their curricula. Medical ethics courses began to be taught in the 1960s, and legal and business ethics classes appeared in the 1970s. The value of these courses is very much in dispute. Some approaches to teaching ethics confuse more than clarify, leaving students with only one distinct impression: There are no absolute principles by which human behavior can be judged. Thus, some of these courses are only exercises in distinguishing allowable (if questionable!) from prosecutable conduct within a given profession.

There are not enough laws, codes of professional ethics, or rules of procedure to compensate for the fundamental lack of personal character among the men and women who practice medicine, argue before the bar, drive taxis, sell clothes, or work in offices. Marilynn Cash Mathews, a former professor at Washington State University, surveyed more than 350 firms and came to the startling and discouraging conclusion that companies with written ethics policies are more often charged with crimes than those without such policies. Rhetoric about "doing good" doesn't translate into ethical professions or companies without something much more fundamental. *It's character, people! Character.*

ETHICAL RELATIVISM

The fact that ethical relativism has dominated American culture during the past quarter century has much to do with our moral state. Ethical relativism takes two forms—individual and cultural. The former claims that ethical judgments are simply forms of saying "I like so-and-so" or "I dislike so-and-so." Moral sentiment is therefore a statement of personal taste toward certain behaviors. The latter holds that ethical judgments mean that culture-specific customs of a certain group have generally approved or disallowed a behavior in question.

Both individual and cultural relativism hold that there are no universal principles binding on all persons but that morality differs from culture to culture and from time to time. Thus all relativists insist that there are no answers to ethical problems that apply intersubjectively (equally binding on all members of a group) or interculturally (equally binding on all cultures). It would appear, then, that the greatest problem for a relativist is to justify even the discussion of morality. Why discuss what cannot be resolved? If discussion must end at the point of personal taste or social rules, why talk about our differences at all?

The very fact that relativists do discuss ethical concerns helps reveal the falsity of their premise about right and wrong. Arguing about a thing implies there is some standard by which the dispute may be resolved. Because there are notoriously difficult cases in ethics, it does not follow that we have learned nothing about appropriate ethical standards over the years. The relativist is guilty of what logicians call "hasty generalization" by reasoning that because individuals and groups *sometimes* disagree about the categorizing of an action as right or wrong, they *always* disagree. They further make the mistake of assuming that there is no way to resolve differences among persons or entities by rational discussion.

The very fact that relativists discuss ethical concerns reveals the falsity of their premise about right and wrong.

An additional fallacy of ethical relativism is its knee-jerk reaction to the idea of identifying ethical principles that are intersubjectively and interculturally correct and useful as the basis for settling disagreements about good and bad behaviors. The alternative to relativism is *not* dogmatism. It is possible to identify core beliefs about human conduct that can serve very much as axioms do for geometry, basic colors for art, or the scale for music. Even for most atheists, the fifth through tenth commandments "make sense" as fundamental moral virtues.

ABSOLUTES *DO* EXIST

We may legitimately claim to have learned some things about the moral life across the centuries. In East and West, among nonreligious and religious people, with formal ethicists and "common folk"—there is an identifiable concurrence of sanctioned moral guidelines (core beliefs, foundational principles) that should be taught people through our institutions, both public and private.

The complexity of some of the social issues of our time (e.g., *in vitro* fertilization, affirmative action, censorship) has given people the wrong idea about ethics generally. Some things *can* be nailed down. There are some things we *know* to be right or wrong. When we move from grand issues of social policy to topics in personal ethics, we can begin to deal with morality in a significant way. Personal ethics is not only more fundamental than social ethics but is also more concrete, objective, and practical. These are the issues addressed in the Ten Commandments.

Russell Gough of the humanities division at Pepperdine University has stated the issue clearly in these words:

> Let's think of personal ethics from now on simply in terms of character. To talk about character is to talk about what kind of person to be, and how to become that kind of person. It is to consider things like respect, honesty, personal responsibility, private decency, and honor. From this angle, ethics becomes very concrete.
>
> The best way for me to explain this point is through examples. Consider: We all agree that we should be the kind of people who, for example, do not mistreat children, do not humiliate people, do not torture animals, do not break promises, do not steal, and do not cheat. We all desire to be the kind of people who avoid these kinds of actions because all of these traits of character are Wrong. No doubt about it.
>
> On the positive side, we all agree that we should be the kind of people who, for example, are considerate

and respectful of others, are charitable and generous, and are fair and honest. We all should be the kind of people who have these traits of character because all of these traits are Right. No doubt about it.

When you consider examples such as these, you begin to sense that the idea of ethics is much, much more than a bunch of gnarly and controversial dilemmas. You can even find examples in social ethics to make the same point. For instance, do we really ever want to say that the sacred notion of human rights is just a matter of opinion? Of course not. There are certain ethical values, social and personal, which transcend mere human opinion. They are as universal as air and as solid as diamonds.

THE UNIQUE RELATIONSHIP OF THE CHRISTIAN TO LAW

People who believe the Bible insist that the best and clearest summary of the moral laws that transcend culture and personal taste are found in the Ten Commandments. We accept them on the basis of our reverence for the God who is their author and, knowing that our salvation is by grace rather than law-keeping, attempt to honor him by living within the parameters of these commands and their underlying principles.

Christian Freedom Leads to Obedience

This life commitment to follow the will of God as revealed in such specific biblical guidance as the Decalogue is the fundamental meaning of Christian discipleship. Men and women in Christ have been set free by him, but we would be incredibly foolish to understand our "freedom" as the freedom to destroy ourselves by self-willed behavior and immorality. To the contrary, we have been set free from the destructiveness of sin so we can live in the freedom of obedience and righteousness.

In the New Testament, Paul affirmed that Christians are "called to be free" (Gal. 5:13a). Knowing the tendency of humans to misinterpret freedom as license, he immediately added: "But do not use your freedom to indulge the sinful nature" (Gal. 5:13b). This is the same tension that modern Christians are still trying to understand, teach, and live.

Salvation Based on Jesus Alone

We accept the wonderful Good News that teaches us that our salvation is a gift from God rather than a reward for our efforts. With Paul, we affirm that rule keeping within a religious system is not the means to salvation. The only ground for salvation we know is the atoning death of Jesus Christ, and we trust his finished work at the cross as the basis of our hope. Our living (submissive, obedient) faith continually reaches to God in gratitude, and our weak (resistant, disobedient) behavior fails to measure up to our desire to honor him.

Relationship with God Maintained by Confession

Ironically, we maintain our fellowship with God not because we have risen above sin but precisely because we confess our sinfulness (1 John 1:9). Thus we have no room for arrogance and smugness before our non-Christian neighbors. We make no hypocritical claim to be better than them. Our claim is a much humbler one that credits a patient and loving God with saving us by his grace. It would be the zenith of human arrogance to claim more. We are not saved because we are good but because he is good.

In our confessional posture as sinners saved by grace, we affirm that God's ways are right and holy. Even when we are deficient in keeping the command about truthfulness, for example, our acknowledgment of that very failure is an affirmation of God's right to demand it of us. Our confession of sin for having failed to be truthful is an admission of the holiness of the commandment that prohibits lying. Paul said as much in Romans 7:13–25.

We maintain our fellowship with God not because we have risen above sin but precisely because we confess our sinfulness.

So Christians are people with a unique relationship to divine law. We do not trust law to save us. Indeed, law makes us painfully aware of our inability to be good enough to deserve salvation, and it prompts us to look to Christ as the only one who can meet our spiritual needs (cf. Gal. 3:22). But we do trust law to give us an insight into God's perfection, point us to the ideal lifestyle that honors him and gives him pleasure, and warn of the land mines in human experience that will destroy us.

AN EMERGING CONSENSUS

Is it possible for us to contribute anything to the public discussion of ethics from our faith perspective? Does the separation of church and state preclude our making a contribution to our schools, communities, and nation as Christians? My response to these questions is that we not only may but must link arms with people of decency and good will from any number of perspectives—atheists, Muslims, Jews, Buddhists—to help improve the moral climate of our world. Religious Bible-believers are not the only ones concerned about morality in our society. The situation has become so desperate that people of every perspective are eager to do something to correct the obvious evils that are doing such harm to our culture.

Cases in Point

Consider a few cases in point. Although I do not endorse such items as abortion on demand that are part of the typical "feminist agenda," it is feminist groups across the United States that are making the most effective argument against pornography: Pornography is rooted in the sexual exploitation of woman; thus it is immoral and ought to be eliminated from mainstream culture. One does not have to subscribe to every element of the feminist platform to work with them in given communities to close peep shows, theaters that specialize in XXX-rated movies, and bookstores that deal in hard-core porn.

In the presidential election of 1992, Republican Dan Quayle was relentlessly castigated as a bigoted buffoon for a speech he made in California. He said:

> Ultimately, however, marriage is a moral issue that requires cultural consensus and the use of social sanctions. Bearing babies irresponsibly is, simply, wrong. . . . It doesn't help matters when prime time TV has Murphy Brown—a character who supposedly epitomizes today's intelligent, highly paid, professional woman—mocking the importance of fathers by bearing a child alone and calling it just another "lifestyle choice."

But the Democratic administration in office after that election—now charged with running the country—began to make "judgmental" statements themselves. Donna Shalala, among the most politically liberal members of the Clinton cabinet, said, "I don't like to put this in moral terms, but I do believe that having children out of wedlock is just wrong." And President Clinton is on record with this: "Would we be a better-off society if babies were born to married couples? You bet we would." Marriage is within the will of God, and the sexual promiscuity that brings about ever increasing rates of illegitimate births is wrong.

We must link arms with people of decency and good will to help improve the moral climate of our world.

As the danger to society becomes more evident, others in the Washington spotlight have witnessed a reversal of attitudes from value-negative sources. Tipper Gore took quite a bashing in the 1980s for her public statements about violent and obscene lyrics in contemporary music. It was trendy for comedians to poke fun at her and for framers of public policy to solemnly explain that First Amendment rights would be violated by the sort of labeling system she proposed. Thus Jesse Jackson defended Sister Souljah's right to rap her lyrics of hatred. Yet the Rainbow Coalition, led by none other than Jesse Jackson, launched an offensive against the record industry in 1994 for its irresponsibility in promoting violence and immorality.

Democrats should help Republicans teach and uphold the integrity of the family, and Republicans should help Democrats. This is not a point of partisan politics but of self-evident truth. Christians of whatever political leaning should applaud anyone in public life who affirms it. They should be able to support any public program that helps strengthen families and willing to oppose any that undermine them.

The mid-term elections of 1994 made the issue of public virtue the central campaign issue across the United States. Setting aside the economy and foreign policy, Republicans and Democrats sounded more like preachers than politicians in some of their campaign ads. "Issues change. Values are constant," said one political analyst. "So it makes sense for a voter to look at somebody's values. That's a critical determinant of their vote." We can only hope that the sound bytes represented real conviction for some of the people who were elected in those campaigns.

According to a front-page story in the *Dallas Morning News* on October 26, 1994, the issue of declining moral values has steadily climbed the list of voter concerns in America. Titled "Moral Commitment," the story cited a recent *Wall Street Journal/NBC News* poll in which 54 percent agreed and 34 percent disagreed that the country's "social problems stem from a decline in moral values rather than financial pressures" on families.

The same article quoted the chairman of the Congressional Black Caucus as pointing to the Ten Commandments with appreciation. "The issue of values cannot be left out of . . . any new commitment to change America, any effort to change communities," said Representative Kweisi Mfume, Democrat from Maryland. "What Moses brought down from Mount Sinai was not the Ten Suggestions, but a blueprint for life."

Defining Right and Wrong

Against the conventional "wisdom" of only a few years ago, there is an emerging consensus that it is possible to formulate, articulate, teach, and demand compliance with a code of ethics in a pluralistic society. The time appears to have come when responsible persons from a variety of backgrounds are willing to unite their influence to say what everyone knows but what many have been too intimidated to say about human behavior: some things are wrong and some things are right, and it is our duty to distinguish between the two.

When such a suggestion is proposed, some protest that an attempt to define right and wrong as objective categories is an attempt to define the details of personal and social ethics for everyone. Not at all! I would resist anyone attempting to do that for me, and I believe all other people have the same fundamental rights I claim for myself. In fact, an understanding of this distinction leads to an understanding of an "ethic of minimal civility" that will allow us to agree upon and enforce a general code of acceptable behavior while still preserving our independence of judgment about the nuances of private and public life. One of the items within such a strategy of moral discussion is respect for personal integrity that renounces the violation of another's autonomy.

AN ETHIC OF MINIMAL CIVILITY

What I have called an *Ethic of Minimal Civility* is not a long list of laws, do-and-don't mandates, and intrusive rules to cover every possible human behavior. It is a statement of foundational ethical principles and basic moral duties that can be applied to particular situations.

There is no claim made here that we can take the Ten Commandments into the marketplace of public discussion and cover every possible type of human behavior and interaction; that is precisely why the use of these principles in the larger culture is called an ethic of *minimal* civility. Its goal is to define a core of right values that can guide ethical decision making. Yet, granting that this is a "minimal" ethic, it is nevertheless helpful enough to guide human behavior toward *civility.* That is, it makes it possible for people to carry on both their private and public lives in respect and dignity. Therein lies the justification for such an ethic—even to those who do not believe the Bible and accept its authority over their lives.

An Ethic of Minimal Civility arises from the principle of mutual respect within the human community.

An Ethic of Minimal Civility arises from the *principle of mutual respect* within the human community. This principle has been expressed in a variety of ways over the centuries of ethical reflection. According to Immanuel Kant, for example, what he called the principle of universalizability is the first principle of moral reasoning. Also called the principle of generalization, it requires us to test behaviors and rules of behavior by attempting to apply them in the same way to all persons. "I am never to act otherwise," Kant wrote, "than so that I could also will that my maxim should become a universal law." Persons must always be treated with respect, not used as means to ends but seen as ends in themselves. Thus, by such a principle, I am led to treat others with fairness and equality. Since we are equally human—whether male or female, Asian or Hispanic, short or tall, exceptionally high IQ or mentally disadvantaged—each of us is obliged to extend to the others of us the same dignity, honor, and respect desired for himself or herself.

If this Kantian principle sounds familiar, it is probably because most of us know the same postulate of morality in a simpler and older form as the Golden Rule. "Do unto others as you would have them do unto you" is the fundamental rule of ethical behavior. Though not derived from Scripture and not dependent on one's belief in God, the universalizability principle parallels the Golden Rule and points to the final six of the Ten Commandments.

Religious Versus Secular

But what about the thorny issue of the relationship between "religious" and "secular" in searching for a common code of ethical behavior in a pluralistic society?

Because of our commitment to the separation of church and state in America, the Ten Commandments are not about to be posted in school classrooms—especially the first four that deal with our responsibilities to God. But Christians can use their influence to incorporate the insights of the Decalogue into the identification of core values that will be championed by boards of education, PTA groups, and teachers as the demand for moral education grows in our society.

Regardless of one's commitment to or disdain for religion in general or for a given faith in particular, centuries of human experience teach us that people from all backgrounds not only *disagree* about some elements of human experience but also *share common ground* on the fundamental tenets of human behavior. For example, every culture—whether religious or nonreligious—has rules against murder and stealing and encourages promise keeping and loyalty.

Teaching the Ethic

How can these rules of conduct best be taught to students and the larger community without violating their autonomy or crossing the boundary that separates moral education from ethical dogmatism? Christina Hoff Sommers, an associate professor of philosophy at Clark University, has made several helpful suggestions in answer to questions of this sort. The four below, with my own added emphasis on the use of Scripture and some suggested nonbiblical resources, summarize her points of primary emphasis.

First, we should acknowledge the responsibility to teach ethics to young people and adults through our public institutions. The method of dealing with ethics for the past quarter century in public education is called "values clarification." It holds that teachers should never give students direct instructions about right and wrong. Leaving children to discover their own values without the benefit of what we have learned over centuries of ethical reflection and experience is comparable to putting them into sophisticated chemistry labs and leaving them to discover their own compounds. While astoundingly positive results *might* come about in such a process, the greater likelihood is that there will be unnecessary injuries and deaths from such a procedure. A telling critique of values clarification and its negative impact on young people has been offered in William

Kilpatrick's *Why Johnny Can't Tell Right from Wrong* (New York: Touchstone Press, 1993).

The myth of value neutrality has helped produce the situation documented by Robert Bellah and his associates in *Habits of the Heart* (Berkeley: University of California Press, 1985). They describe American culture as one in which people are so enmeshed in individualism that they have no way to make moral sense of their lives. Without a vision of something larger than individual relativism, we all become selfish islands to ourselves.

Second, we should formulate behavior codes for classroom and marketplace that emphasize civility. Cheating will not be tolerated, not because the teacher doesn't like it (has no personal taste for it), but because it is wrong. False advertising will not be countenanced, not because it might "backfire" on the company if discovered, but because lying is wrong. Why cheating, lying, and other behaviors are wrong will be made intelligible by publicly agreed upon behavior codes that have been adopted, published for students and teachers, and followed with consistency.

Third, those who lead this process must refuse to be intimidated by the ill-informed cry that having and observing reasonable codes of behavior is "brainwashing." To the contrary, brainwashing is a process that diminishes someone's ability to think and come to reasoned conclusions. Good moral habits of telling the truth, respecting the property and rights of others, and keeping one's word empower ethical decision making. Without someone teaching a student the plain facts of vocabulary, syntax, and grammar, the likelihood that she will ever write well is severely diminished. Without someone teaching a student the plain facts of truthfulness, autonomy, and justice, the likelihood that she will behave responsibly within her society is greatly reduced.

Fourth, we can adopt a methodology that relies more on positive stories that teach positive ethical principles than the current method of simply offering moral dilemmas for discussion. Children are not prepared to form opinions about euthanasia and foreign policy until they have acquired certain fundamental notions of the moral life. Our recent practice of putting them into these debates where exceptional circumstances and razor-sharp distinctions are the rule undermines their confidence that there is anything that may be called "right" or "wrong" in moral terms. The decision about removing a comatose person from life-support devices is complex in a way that cheating on a math test is not. The issue of abortion in cases of rape and incest is intricate in its details and implications in a way that stealing from one's employer is not.

Every culture preserves stories—whether through fables or about real-life characters—that transmit fundamental values about honesty, fair treatment of others, and courage. William Bennett's *The Book of Virtues* (New York: Simon & Schuster, 1993) is an excellent collection of great moral stories selected from a wide range of sources, appropriate for reading at various age levels, and grouped around the following ten virtues: self-discipline, compassion, responsibility, friendship, work, courage, perseverance, honesty, loyalty, and faith. Also, Kilpatrick's *Why Johnny Can't Tell Right from Wrong* contains an annotated guide to more than 120 books for children and young adults that are valuable to the process of moral education. There are biographies of Abraham Lincoln, Thomas Edison, Susan B. Anthony, Martin Luther King Jr., and others that can be read with moral benefit. Eventually there will be time to read

Plato's *Apology,* Tolstoy's *Death of Ivan Ilych,* and Harper Lee's *To Kill a Mockingbird.*

For Christians, of course, the best single source of both ethical principles and stories that reinforce them will always be the Bible. There are no better examples of virtue than the ones found in the biblical accounts of Noah and the Ark, David and Goliath, Joseph in Egypt, and the life of Jesus. The value of having solid, Bible-teaching programs in local churches where, from pulpits and in Bible study groups, the Word of God is taught faithfully probably doesn't need to be argued to people who would read this volume. Family and personal time with Scripture are needed in addition to church and study group experiences. We must saturate ourselves with the truth of God in order to remain "unspotted by the world" and to justify our behavior to those who question it.

The distinctive elements of Christian morality move ethics to a *maximal* level.

The Christian's *Maximal* Level of Ethics

The justification Christians offer for many of their behaviors will parallel that given by non-Christians. Stealing, lying, breaking promises—these are not only forbidden in the Bible but defy what has been called an Ethic of Minimal Civility. Paul tied this phenomenon of shared moral principles between Jews and Gentiles to the fact that "Gentiles, even though they do not have the law," still sometimes live in such a way that "they show that the requirements of the law are written on their hearts" (Rom. 2:14–15). The distinctive elements of Christian morality, elements that move ethics to a *maximal* level, are derived directly from the theistic commitment they embrace. The call to pursue the perfection of our heavenly Father (cf. Matt. 5:48) or to imitate certain attitudes and behaviors of Jesus (cf. Phil. 2:5 ff.) are distinctive to believers.

CONCLUSION

As long ago as 1966, John Neitz, professor of education at the University of Pittsburgh, found that before 1776, religion and ethics accounted for more than 90 percent of the content of school readers. By 1926 this figure had declined to six percent, and in more recent times had become too small to be measured. It was his thesis that the decline in morality and rise of crime being witnessed in the '60s was traceable to this shift away from moral instruction. Comparing the content of the McGuffey Readers, which were saturated with character-building stories of the sort recommended in this chapter for teaching ethics, and more recent multicultural, "politically correct" literature now given children to read in schools is simultaneously revealing and depressing. The children given the latter "value-neutral" literature are the adolescent and young adult populations who strike terror in the hearts of law-abiding citizens.

In a radio address by President Clinton in December of 1993, this was offered: "Let's face it, drugs and guns and violence fill a vacuum where the values of civilized life used to be." He continued and pressed the point that all Americans have an obligation to "fight violence with values." Would that this theme become the marching orders of a nation for the next generation.

"Whether we're ministers or moviemakers, business people or broadcasters, teachers or parents," he continued, "we can all set our sons and daughters on a better path in life." And the best place to begin that process is with a return to the ethical guidelines that were written in stone by Yahweh 3,500 years ago when he met with Moses on the mountain. May God write these principles on our hearts, give us the wisdom to embrace his righteous will, and enable his people to be salt and light in America before we learn the full meaning of the disgrace sin brings to a nation.

The issue is character, my friend. Character.

QUESTIONS FOR ADDITIONAL REFLECTION

1. Does a written ethics policy guarantee ethical behavior in a company or profession? What is the benefit, if any, of having such guidelines? Are there liabilities?

2. All of us occasionally "link arms" with people from other religious traditions and even nonreligious people to address issues (e.g., combating pornography or providing disaster relief). What benefits come from such efforts?

3. Are there negatives or dangers in these joint efforts with people from dissimilar backgrounds? If so, identify some of them and explain how to deal with them.

4. What does the word *discipleship* mean? What is a Christian's fundamental responsibility with regard to his or her behavior?
5. Does Christian discipleship contradict human freedom? Explain the things Paul said about freedom in Galatians.
6. What is ethical relativism? In what ways have you encountered this spirit in your community?
7. What is the problem with allowing people to "discover their own values"?
8. What stories do you know that you could recommend for the moral instruction of children? Explain your choices by identifying the ethical principle embodied in each story.
9. What is "value-neutral literature"? Does such literature really exist? Why or why not?
10. How can your church be more involved in influencing the character of people in the community where you live?